Fools and Mad

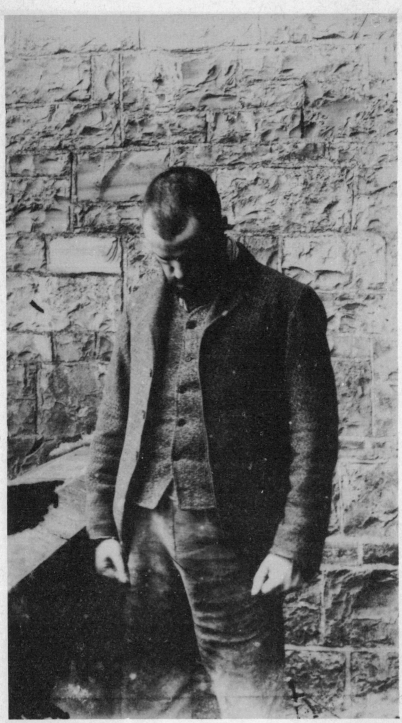

'... an air of bleakness and desolation more calculated to fix than to remove the awful disease ...' (*p. 132*)

Fools and Mad

A HISTORY OF THE INSANE
IN IRELAND

Joseph Robins

INSTITUTE OF PUBLIC ADMINISTRATION

First published 1986

by the Institute of Public Administration
57-61 Lansdowne Road, Dublin 4, Ireland

© Joseph Robins, 1986
    author of *The Lost Children: A Study of Charity Children in Ireland
    1700–1900*

ISBN 0 906980 46 1

British Library Cataloguing in Publication Data

Robins, Joseph
    Fools and mad.
    1. Mentally ill — Care and treatment — Ireland
    — History
    I. Title
    362.2'90415   RC 450.173

Jacket design and layout of photographs, Gene Lambert
Typeset by Print Prep, Dublin
Printed by Brough, Cox and Dunn Limited, Belfast.

TO THE MEMORY OF MY PARENTS

He gave the little Wealth he had
To build a House for Fools and Mad
And shew'd by one satyric Touch
No Nation wanted it so much

'Verses on the Death of Dr Swift'
Jonathan Swift, 1731

Contents

ACKNOWLEDGEMENTS

Permission to reproduce the plates following page 152, the frontispiece and dust-jacket photograph, and the endpaper drawings is gratefully acknowledged; to the library, Trinity College, Dublin for the plates from an early edition of Swift's *Tale of a Tub,* Charles Bell's *Essays on the Anatomy of the Expression in Painting,* 'Taking lunatics to Dublin in the early part of the 19th century', of the, 'circulating swing'; to the National Library of Ireland for the, '19th century continental image of drunken Irish peasants'; to the State Paper Office, Dublin for the Richmond Lunatic Asylum affidavit and medical certificate; to the Midland Health Board and St Loman's Hospital, Mullingar for the plates captioned, 'Moral treatment...', 'Inmates of a district lunatic asylum, late 19th century', '...overall there was a preponderance of males...', 'Images of Irish insanity, late 19th century', 'Prominent asylum doctors, 1892'; to the O'Brien Press for the part elevation of St Columba's Hospital, Sligo which first appeared in *Buildings of Irish Towns;* to Maura and Patrick Shaffrey for the plan of St Columba's Hospital, Sligo; to the Royal College of Surgeons in Ireland for the picture of Dr Francis White; to the Western Health and Social Services Board, Omagh for the pictures of Dr Francis West, 19th century and asylum governors, and for the timetable for winter months, Omagh District Asylum, 1916; to the Philadelphia Museum of Art for the lithograph by George Bellows, 'Dance in a Madhouse' from the ARS MEDICA: Art, Medicine and the Human Condition Collection, made possible by SmithKline Beckman Corporation; to the South Eastern Health Board and St Luke's Hospital, Clonmel for the photograph of Clonmel asylum staff on strike, 1919.

Foreword

My primary aim in compiling this history has been to provide an account of the position of mentally afflicted persons in Ireland in the past. It will, I hope, also serve as a reminder of the way society has for so long mistreated them and contribute to the removal of the vestiges of prejudice and discrimination.

It seemed to me that the early 1960s was an appropriate time to terminate the account. These years marked the end of an era as the care of the mentally ill started moving rapidly away from the attitudes and methods of the past. In any event it would have been difficult for me as a serving public servant to comment freely and objectively on later developments since I had some official association with them. The epilogue summarises very briefly the main features of these later years; and the bibliography includes references to the more recent legislation and relevant government reports. Since it might be confusing I have not attempted to describe the separate development of the Northern Ireland services since 1922; but I have listed the main sources of information for that period in the bibliography.

I have had some difficulty throughout the book in regard to terminology such as the use of the words lunacy, insanity, lunatic, madman and fool. Some of the sources drawn upon used them in a broad generic sense; others applied them to specific groups; some were ambiguous. I have done my best to interpret correctly what was intended. I have also tried throughout to use the terminology current during the period

1

being described. While modern terms would have sounded more sensitive they would have failed to convey the historical aura.

I am thankful to Professor John Jackson (Trinity College, Dublin) for reading a draft of the book and for making valuable suggestions about it. Dr Dermot Walsh (Medico-Social Research Board) gave me helpful comments on statistical trends. Dr Rolf Baumgarten (Dublin Institute for Advanced Studies) provided me with valuable references to insanity in early Irish scripts. The governors of St Patrick's Hospital allowed me access to their eighteenth century records. Alan Gilbert (Department of Health and Social Services, Belfast) helped me in regard to material about Northern Ireland. Professor John McKenna gave me a copy of Dr Louis Clifford's unpublished report of 1943 on his investigation of the incidence of mental handicap. Donal O'Sullivan (Southern Health Board) let me see Daniel Murphy's unpublished historical account of the psychiatric nursing staff of Our Lady's Hospital, Cork.

I wish also to acknowledge the help in various ways of Rev Professor Donal Kerr (St Patrick's College, Maynooth); Dr Eoin O'Brien, Eamonn Ó hOgain (Royal Irish Academy); Dr Seamus Ó Cathain (Department of Irish Folklore, UCD); Donal Ó Luanaigh (National Library); Mary Monahan (Donegal County Library); Peter McQuillan (South Eastern Health Board); Rev Professor F.X. Martin (University College Dublin); Kathleen Keane (An Bord Altranais); Ruth Barrington (Department of Health); Donal Murphy (Nenagh); Dr H. Jocelyn Eustace; Dr Patrick Power (Ennis); Dr Michael Mulcahy and David Devine (Stewart's Hospital); Tom Daly (North Western Health Board); Eamonn Lonergan (St Luke's Hosptial, Clonmel); Rev Professor Martin McNamara (Milltown Institute); Reginald Crampton (St Patrick's Hospital); Robert McCullagh; James Harney and John Clarke (St Loman's Hospital, Mullingar); Robert McKinley (Tyrone and Fermanagh Hospital, Omagh); my sons Eunan and Killian; the keeper and staff of the Public Record Office; the library staffs of Trinity College, Dublin; National Library

Dublin; Royal Irish Academy; Royal College of Physicians of Ireland and the Medical School, Queen's University, Belfast. I also thank the honorary librarian of the Society of Friends, Dublin.

Finally, I am grateful to Patricia Hamill who had the difficult task of deciphering and typing my script.

J. R.

Struck by the Madman's Wisp

In early times all illness was believed to be supernatural in origin; when it came it was due to the malignant influence of some deity. It could hardly have been otherwise in a simple, unscientific society with an unswerving belief that all good and all evil were divinely inspired. Illness was the penalty paid for wrong-doing, for offending a deity or some pagan priest armed with powerful and terrible rites and incantations. The cure, like the cause, could usually be found only in further supernatural intervention when the wrath of the gods had been appeased.

The advent of Christianity changed little. It simply put a Christian gloss on existing notions particularly in isolated communities like Ireland where many of the beliefs about the origins and treatment of illness remained rooted for centuries mainly in pagan beliefs. Furthermore, while the more rational but largely erroneous concepts of medicine put forward by early doctors like Hippocrates, Galen and Celsus were for many centuries to influence medical thinking, they made little impact on relatively primitive people like the Irish who were peripheral to the Greek and Roman cultures from which these ideas had emerged. One of the first entries in the *Annals of the Four Masters* is an indication of the contemporary beliefs about physical illness. It records that in 1171AD Dermot MacMurrogh, King of Leinster:

became, putrid while living by the miracles of God,

through the intervention of Columcille, Finnen and other saints of Ireland for having violated and burned their churches[1].

If there were any doubts about the origins of physical illness there were none where insanity was concerned. Faced with strange, irrational and disturbed behaviour, early society, in the absence of any other explanation, could see in it only the hand of God or possession by some evil spirit. *Deuteronomy,* dating from the seventh century BC and reflecting current beliefs, contains a warning by Moses to his people that if they 'will not obey the voice of the Lord your God or be careful to do all his commandments and his statutes . . . the Lord will smite you with madness and blindness and confusion of mind'. The Greeks regarded mental derangement as a form of punishment by the gods and the later Roman civilisation took a similar view[2].

It was a view that was to prevail for centuries varying only in detail according to local cultural and religious influences. Where Ireland was concerned the Brehon laws, the old legends and later folklore all reflect a continuing belief in the supernatural origin of insanity.

The madman's wisp

In pre-Christian Ireland one of the most dreaded powers attributed to the highly respected and greatly feared Druidic priests was that of causing madness. A Druid prepared a 'madman's wisp', a ball of straw or grass, and was believed to produce madness by throwing it in the victim's face. The invention of the wisp is attributed to a celebrated Leinster Druid, Fullon, who lived centuries before the Christian era[3]. Belief in it prevailed at least until early in the fifth century AD when the *Senchus Mór,* containing the codified laws of ancient Ireland, was compiled. This important source of information about the early Irish refers repeatedly to a madman as one upon whom the *dlui fulla* or Fullon's wisp had been thrown. Since the *Senchus* dates from a period when Christianity was yet in the process of being established in Ireland its concept of the origin of madness was still rooted in Druidic beliefs. As already pointed out little changed under the early Christian influence; mental derangement continued to have its origins in some malign supernatural force. An incident involving St Mochuda reflects that view. Mochuda was visited by a man who was mad 'owing to a demon having entered into him'; he interceded with God and the man was cured. In a later period a Norman archer was reputed to have been struck mad because he entered a forbidden area surrounding an ever-burning fire at Kildare believed to have been lit originally by St Brigid[4].

The madness of battle
Throughout Irish mythology and particularly in the Ossianic legends there are references to a type of madness induced by the frenzy of battle. Warriors crazed by the carnage around them became light as air and rising up like birds fled the battle-field. During the battle of Ventry which lasted for a year and a day between Dara Donnmar, 'the Monarch of the World', and the warriors of Ireland it is related of Vulcan, the King of France:

> ... there came lightness of mind and of nature upon him and he gave his body a stretching from the ground so that he went with the wind and the madness before the eyes of the hosts of the world and did not stop until he came to Gleann Bolcain in the east of that territory[5].

During the second battle of Moytura it is said that the chief druid of Nuada, King of the Dedannan, rushed from the conflict 'in madness and red lunacy'[6]. According to one translation of an account of the battle of Allen in 772 AD 'there were nine persons that flyed in the air as if they were winged fowle'; elsewhere they are referred to as 'nine ferocious flying madmen'[7]. William Camden, the English historian and antiquary, writing towards the end of the sixteenth century, claimed that this belief in flying madmen was then still current among the 'wild Irish'[8].

The most famous of these demented warriors was Mad Sweeney *(Suibhne Geilt)* who fled the battle of Moyrath in 637 AD and about whom a long and moving epic tale, *Buile Suibhne,* was written in about the twelfth century. It relates how Sweeney, a local chieftain, was cursed by Ronan the Fair, abbot of Drumiskin, following a dispute over the site of a church. Ronan's imprecation condemned Sweeney to a life wandering and flying through the world until speared to death. Some time later Sweeney takes part in the battle of Moyrath where, maddened by the slaughter, he rises in the air and flies to the same glen in which Vulcan had previously sought peace. He continues to wander fluttering from tree-top to tree-top pursued for a time by a hag.

He has strange and terrifying Bosch-like visions which reflect his demented state. At midnight on Slieve Mish he sees:

> ... trunks, headless and red, and heads without bodies, and five bristling rough grey heads without body or trunk among them, screaming and leaping this way and that about the world.

They pursue him shrieking and clutching at him until he escapes 'into the filmy clouds of the sky'. His wanderings subsequently take him to Britain where he becomes friendly with another madman, Ealadhan, but he eventually returns to Ireland and joins a community attached to St Moling. Here, in keeping with Ronan's curse, he is speared to death by a swineherd who has accused him of adultery with his wife[9].

Early terminology

The terminology of insanity in the early Irish legal manuscripts and the later glossaries associated with them provide some clues to contemporary notions on the different types of mental abnormality. There was, however, a profusion of terms, some of them used inconsistently, and Gaelic scholars have had difficulty in establishing their exact meaning. The following summary does not, therefore, contain all the descriptive terms used in the old texts, or the different interpretations of them.

The name for a fool was *drúth*. He appears to have been invested with Divine protection for he is described as *co rath Dé*, 'with the grace of God'. This is probably the origin of the modern Irish phrase *duine le Dia*, 'person of God' and is close to *enfant Dieu* in use on the continent in medieval and later times. It was used to distinguish the fool (usually a congenitally handicapped person) from the madman so long regarded as a manifestation of evil.

According to one text there were three broad classifications of *drúth* which were in turn sub-classified. Firstly there were 'fools with talent' including the *bobre* ('having the behaviour of the cow'), the *biocmell* ('under whose neck are the soft lumps'), the *righ drúth* ('the king fool'), the *mellach suirig* and the *rindineach*. The second group consisted of 'persons of half sense' which included the *buice* ('who has the mist on his head'), the *finelogh* ('half foolish and half wise') and the *caeptha*. The remaining group represented 'the madman without talent' and included the *saluch drúth* ('the unclean fool') [10]. It has not been possible to give a translation for some of these names as there is uncertainty about their meaning. Subsequently *óinmhid* came to be used to describe a fool of either sex and this was replaced in later Irish by *óinseach* for a female and *amadán* for a male [11].

As well as the various classifications of *drúth* the ancient laws refer to two other categories of insane persons, the *mer* and the *dásachtach*. The *mer* is translated into English as 'idiot' and is described as 'one without grace'. The *dásachtach* is translated as 'lunatic' or 'madman' and is invariably described as one on whom the magic wisp has been thrown [12].

In some of the earliest Gaelic poems and legends the word *geilt* is used both as a noun and an adjective to describe a madman and *geltacht* to describe the state of madness. The earliest use of *geilt* is to be found in poetry believed to date from the eighth or ninth century. A quarrel between Finn and his son Oisin described in a poem from that period has Oisin abusively describing his father as a *geilt*. The word is also to be found in other works of the period and has been used in particular to describe those who went mad in battle[13]. It is now often spelt as *gealt*. Despite a similarity to *gealac*, the word for 'moon', Gaelic scholars have no evidence of any etymological connection between them.

It is not possible with certainty to relate any of the foregoing descriptions to the modern classification of the mentally afflicted. Those translated as 'idiots' and 'fools' were probably in the main congenitally abnormal individuals who would today be classified as mentally handicapped while the 'lunatics' and 'madpersons' would probably now be regarded as mentally ill. But it is possible only to speculate; centuries were to elapse before clear distinctions were established.

The moon and madness

From the earliest times there was a universal belief that the moon caused madness. In Ireland it can be traced to the pre-Christian period when the moon was the object of worship under the name of Aine or Anu. In Dunany (Co. Louth) a large rock on the sea-shore called Cathaoir Ana (the Madman's Chair) was popularly believed to have been named after the moon although one account ascribed the name to a female fairy. It was said that insane persons drawn by some irresistible impulse made their way to it and seated themselves thrice on it. This, according to one source, could cure their malady. Sane persons sitting on it ran the risk of losing their senses. Another account suggests that unless the insane person sat on the rock during a recession in his illness he would not be cured, since the effect of the rock was to stabilise for life the degree of sanity or insanity he possessed prior to sitting on it. Rabid dogs from all over the country were also said to be lured to the rock by the same strange force and then, retreating from it, to swim out to their deaths in the sea as the impulse drew them to Aine's underwater kingdom[14]. Belief in the power of the moon persisted down through the centuries. An English visitor describing Irish customs in 1691 wrote:

When they first see the moon after the change commonly they bow the knee and say the Lord's prayer and then speak to the moon 'leave us as whole and as sound as thou has found us'[15].

This respect survives in the folklore of rural Ireland collected in the 1930-50 period. In Kerry it was believed that those born at the time of a 'castrated moon' (*ré caoillte*) would suffer misfortune and that madness reached its peak when the moon was full. In Galway a 'sandy moon' was blamed for causing many persons to lose their mind[16].

The glen of the mad

There are few more fascinating features in the folklore and mythology of the insane in Ireland than the beliefs which grew up over a period of centuries in regard to Glannagalt (the glen of the mad) in County Kerry. This beautiful valley in the shadow of the mountains near Castlegregory figures frequently in the folklore of Kerry and in various legends of ancient Ireland as a place to which insane persons were irresistibly drawn. While there are no specific references to it before 1584 a modern study of the old Gaelic texts describing the glen to which the berserk Vulcan fled from the battle of Ventry and Mad Sweeney from the battle of Moyrath leaves little doubt that the location was the valley later to be known as Glannagalt[17]. This suggests that there was belief in the strange healing powers of the glen as early as the twelfth century when the first of these texts was composed. It was a belief that broadened and strengthened with the years. By the eighteenth century it was widely thought that if no obstacle were placed in their way all the insane persons of Ireland would be drawn to the valley. There at Ahagoltaun (the madman's ford) they would cross the stream which flows through the valley and passing by Clocnagalt (the madman's stone) would eat watercress and drink from Tobarnagalt (the madman's well). The description of the ritual varies in detail in different accounts but not to any substantial degree. The hoped-for outcome of the journey was that the strange powers of the glen would restore the sanity of the insane person[18].

For a considerable period these sad demented wanderers were a common sight in the area. Almost certainly many of them were taken there and abandoned by their families in the simple-minded hope that they would eventually return home cured. Friar O'Sullivan of Muckross Abbey, writing about 1750, described some of them as 'dumb, very hairy, with dismall and ruefull looks'[19]. Later reports describe cures believed to have taken place. They include that of Mary Maher who came to the glen 'rabidly mad and entirely naked' in 1823 and went home sane in mind; and a man named Sullivan who in 1839 returned 'entirely cured of his lunacy in three days'[20].

According to various folk stories of the Munster counties it was not unusual for lovers who lost their minds as a result of being jilted to seek solace in the glen. In an old Gaelic love poem, *Cuirim céad slán chun Dun Gharbháin* a heart-broken lover laments:

> *A Rí na bFheart go reidhir ár nglas*
> *Agus go gceangalair sinn le na chéile*
> *Nó raghad gan stad go Gleann na nGealt*
> *Mora bhfagaidh me tú mar céile*[21] .

With the development of a system of district lunatic asylums during the nineteenth century popular belief in the mysterious curative qualities of the glen gradually faded. It was understandable that the superstitions of centuries should give way in the face of the care and prospects of cure that the new asylums had to offer. One of these asylums was established locally in Killarney. It soon became evident that the changed attitudes were to influence not only the insane and their families. The long suffering inhabitants of the Glannagalt area had always feared their visitors and many had placed protective bars on the windows of their homes. If they had previously shown tolerance towards the strange disturbed persons wandering their roads and living in their hedges and woods it was probably out of a combination of Christian charity and the timorous regard which Irish peasants in general had for deeply rooted superstitions. Now with the establishment of

11

the asylum in Killarney they no longer felt an obligation to submit passively to harassment by wandering lunatics. A resistance, sometimes violent, to them gradually developed. One account describes how a naked lunatic from the North was shot at by a local inhabitant named Falvey and was so frightened that he was restored to his senses. According to local folklore the shooting by a local farmer of another wanderer found stealing milk from a cow led to an exodus from the area while a further account describes the local people acting *en masse* to drive the lunatics away. By the 1880s the resistance of the local population had finally quenched the belief in the strange powers of their glen and it was restored to a tranquillity that it had not known for centuries[22].

Other centres of pilgrimage

Other surviving centres of pilgrimage for the insane were largely local in character; there were several such places in Donegal. There was a well at Port a Doruis near Inishowen Head to which all the madmen of the area were said to be attracted. They also congregated at a stream, Sruv Broin (the stream of sorrow), in Moville parish[23]. Not far away near Malin Head there was a small hollow in a rock, referred to by one source as Cloc na Madaidh, which filled with sea water at every tide and was reputed to possess the power of curing disease, particularly madness. It attracted more than the mad. A report written in 1816 said that 'strollers and mendicants of the worse description from the three adjoining counties . . . infest the neighbourhood by their numbers and corrupt it by their example'. The Church refused to acknowledge the existence of the patron of the rock, Saint Moriallagh, and condemned 'the most disgusting drunkenness and debauchery' associated with it. Not surprisingly the local population was fearful of many of the visitors. A later account describes the people in Malin parish building their homes close together 'because of the threat of rambling mad-men'. At the same time there was some compassion for the insane pilgrims and they were often given shelter for the night if not regarded as dangerous[24]. Yet another Donegal location associated with the cure of insanity as well as other illness was Saint Conal's Well near the village of Bruckless. It is of interest that the local district mental hospital in Letterkenny is called St Conal's Hospital[25].

There were many holy wells throughout Ireland not specifically associated with the cure of insanity which attracted the sick in general. Some still survive. Other wells were visited not for their religious associations but because they were spa wells rich in minerals such as iron or sulphur. Some of these were to be found in the Leitrim and Cavan area. It is possible, for example, that persons depressed as a result of iron deficiency anaemia benefited from drinking the water. Furthermore, as far as holy and spa wells in general were concerned, it is probable that belief in their powers may have had the same effect as good psychotherapy[26].

Kilbarry in County Roscommon on the shores of Lough Forbes had a centre of pilgrimage for the insane which was somewhat different from those already described. In ruins believed to be the sixth century oratory of St Barry insane persons and their friends kept vigil for several days and nights. The requirements were that the sick person should pass the nights of Thursday, Friday and Saturday in the ruins and should attend Mass in Kilbarry on Sunday morning. According to Logan *(The Holy Wells of Ireland)*, it was a hopeful sign if he slept throughout the three nights but even if he did not sleep the miraculous influence of the ruins could bring some relief[27].

A traveller on the Shannon in 1852 who had visited the ruins described seeing a patient lying on straw as his relatives huddled around the watchfire in the chilly night. They were, he wrote:

> ... roughly clad men, gaunt and brown as the surrounding bog passing the glass from one to another ... watching anxiously with their women[28].

As an image it serves to sum up the attitude of a simpler society faced with the strange and incomprehensible affliction of insanity.

Protection and Persecution

The belief of the early Irish that insanity had supernatural origins did nothing to diminish the reality of its existence nor the social issues it could create. It was a phenomenon they recognised in a rational and pragmatic way when eventually they came to regulate the society in which they lived. The Brehon laws, that remarkable body of ancient laws of Ireland which developed during the pre-Christian and early Christian period and had force until Elizabethan times, contained considerable provision for the insane. In general they were admirable provisions which, as long as they operated, provided wide legal protection for the insane in Ireland.

The Brehon laws
The laws distinguished broadly between idiots, fools and lunatics but frequently sub-classified each group in designating their legal rights and obligations. These classifications have been referred to earlier *see* page 8. A major influence on the classifications appears to have been the extent to which the individual was adjudged capable of work or had the potential for being amusing or otherwise useful.

The numerous legal provisions ranged between those relating to the insane in general and those concerning specific groups. It was decided at the end of seven years of age if a person were a fool or a sensible person. If a fool inherited land it was kept undivided for a period of five successive occupants and if at the end of a hundred years a sensible son

14

should be descended from the fool the land was handed over to him. Contracts were not binding on any insane persons unless authorised by their guardians at the time they were made. However the contract of a fool or of a madwoman was invalid even if the latter condition were met. Fools and madmen were exempted from the penalties for wrongdoing but in the case of fools those responsible for their care were obliged to compensate the injured party. Where a person of 'half reason or sense' committed a crime, responsibility for compensation was imposed on the father or mother or 'the stranger who lodges in the house'.

Where a person failed to provide for the maintenance of a fool who had some land as well as 'the power of amusing' there was a fine of five cows. On the other hand the fine for not maintaining a madwoman was ten cows because a madwoman could neither be a minstrel nor have land. A fool without land or the capacity to amuse was regarded as in a similar category[2].

There was a variety of other forms of protection. Where a madman and a madwoman had been encouraged to have sexual intercourse by persons making fun of them, the persons concerned were obliged to foster any consequent offspring and were also responsible for the crimes of such offspring. A fool taken to assist in stealing cattle was freed from responsibility. The owner of a dog had an obligation to prevent him attacking an insane person; the guardian of such a person was in turn required to prevent him from provoking dogs. If a fool was set drunk in an ale house those who brought him there or those who served him became responsible for any consequent misdeeds he might commit. The laws distinguished between the intoxication of drunkenness (*meisce lenna*) and the intoxication of madness (*meisce merachta*)[3].

Figures of fun

Apart from legal protection there is no evidence that special arrangements of any significance for the insane existed in Ireland prior to the eighteenth century. On the basis of the Brehon laws and the limited information available from other sources it is clear that insane persons were normally looked after by their family or tribe. Some of them were figures of fun and, as the laws indicate, it was legitimate to employ them for amusement purposes so long as they were given adequate care. This was not a uniquely Irish attitude; the fool had been mocked from earliest times but particularly so throughout medieval and Renaissance Europe. So, too, were some of the physically disabled[4].

The Pharoahs of ancient Egypt loved to surround themselves with ugly dwarfs and in the Roman Empire human freaks and monstrosities were exposed for sale in the market place[5]. In Irish legend it is related that Finn McCool had a tiny harper — a dwarf named Cnú Deireoil — who was said to be the best harper in Ireland[6]. This story might suggest that early Irish society also valued physical abnormality.

But the greatest demand was for the more striking and amusing manifestations of imbecility. Court fools were kept in the royal courts of Britain and France during medieval times and great importance was attached to their capacity to entertain at court festivities. They may not always have been mad, however, and a distinction was drawn as early as the twelfth century between 'natural' fools and 'artificial' fools, the latter being the equivalent of the professional clown of modern society. Fools and human freaks were also familiar figures of the social life of the Renaissance period. In 1580 Lucrezia Borgia gave a banquet at which two dwarfs were served up with the fruit to amuse the ladies. The French and Spanish courts exchanged fools and Velasquez recorded for posterity the infinitely sad faces of some of the dwarf entertainers of Spanish royalty. In Britain the Stuart kings, like their continental brethren, kept a retinue of dwarfs and fools. By the eighteenth century the institution of the court fool was fading everywhere except in some backward countries like Russia[7].

Monastic provisions
It is not clear to what extent the Irish monastic system cared for the insane. Since their custody was normally regarded as

the responsibility of relatives and friends it was almost certainly on a small scale. In general, monasteries throughout medieval Europe cared only for a small number of the more troublesome insane by locking them in cells and it is reasonable to assume that the same practice was adopted in Ireland. Tuke interprets references in some medieval accounts, including that of Giraldus Cambrensis, the Welsh monk who spent a period in Ireland towards the end of the twelfth century, as indicating that the insane in these islands were sometimes kept in fetters and chains in the monasteries[8].

The notable lack of references to the insane in the extant records of Irish monastic centres can be regarded as confirming that these did not provide for them in any special way or to any significant degree. It is almost certain, however, that from time to time they were given food and shelter by the monasteries because they were regarded as wayfarers. There were always deranged persons who had been cast adrift by their families; the wandering madman, or 'the lunatic at large' as he came to be known by the eighteenth century, was a fairly common feature of Irish society over a considerable period of time. Hospitality to the poor and to the wayfarer was an essential element of Irish monastic life as it was elsewhere. There was a considerable range of hospitals and hospices in medieval Ireland operated by the Knights Hospitallers and by the regular religious orders such as the Benedictines, Augustinians and Trinitarians[9]. In general the amount of accommodation provided in them for sick and infirm persons appears to have been quite small. A hospital associated with the Cistercian monastery in Cashel, one of the largest monasteries, had towards the end of the thirteenth century only fourteen beds[10].

With the closure of the monasteries as the Reformation developed during the sixteenth century the main provision for the sick and poor disappeared. Those seeking help had nowhere to turn. At least one Irish lunatic, so described in British state papers, wrote to Queen Elizabeth about 1587. He was Roger Crymble, clearly a literate and imaginative man:

You are placed by Christ in the Paradyce as Adam was in the beginning, to dresse the garden, to pull up the weeds, to cherish the good herbs that when God in the cool of day doth come to walk therein he may find all things well. And now my good mistress Gardener where shall the Crymbles growe so that this cold wynter the frost may not kill them considering we are some of the sweet smelling flowers unto God . . .[11].

Witchcraft and madness

For a considerable period church and state throughout Europe pursued the so-called crime of witchcraft with a manic determination; huge numbers of alleged witches were put to death with considerable cruelty. Many of them were insane persons.

From early Christian times belief in witches and occult practices was regarded as sinful and condemned by the Church. An early synod of the Irish Church dating from about 457 AD denounced Christians who believed in the existence of *lamias* and *strigae*, the night-flying, blood-sucking demons who were part of the pagan demonology. Such beliefs were also condemned in the later penitential books intended for the guidance of the clergy which described sins in detail and established appropriate penances for them. The sin of witchcraft in particular was dealt with in the Penetential of Columba originating in Ireland about 600 AD[12].

Yet, while the early Christian Church condemned witchcraft its practice was regarded with a certain degree of tolerance; it was seen merely as a fading survival of paganism. But if it was considered to pose no threat to a united Church such was not the case as the first heresies spread, as rival popes emerged and as the terrible ravages of the Black Death gave rise to a less settled society. Gradually those believed to be witches came to be regarded as the representatives of the evil and satanic influences threatening the integrity of the Church. Both the illiterate majority and the intellectual *élite* considered them to be involved in such activies as promiscuous and incestuous nocturnal orgies presided over by the Devil in the form of an animal, usually a cat. They were believed to concoct diabolic potions, to burn babies and to cast dreadful spells. These demonological fantasies came to be associated with heretics. While some so-called witches were not involved in heresy, others were. Witchcraft, for some, had become a cult, an extreme form of social revolt against the dominant religion of the period[13].

By the end of the thirteenth century all heretics were subject to harsh punishment, including death, throughout the Christian countries. In the fourteenth century a Bull issued by Pope John XXII left no doubt about the Church's attitude to witchcraft, in particular, and in the following century Innocent VIII launched an even more vigorous crusade. This culminated in the publication in 1489 by two German inquisitors of *Malleus Maleficarum* (The Hammer of the Witches), the famous text book on procedure in witch-craft cases. Men, women and children were condemned as witches. It is of interest that the tendency to find more witches among women possibly originated with the views expressed in the German text book that witchcraft was more natural to women because of the inherent wickedness of their hearts[14].

Following the Reformation the persecution of witchcraft was adopted by the Protestant reformers with even greater zeal than its Catholic begetters. In the sixteenth and seventeenth centuries thousands of unfortunate persons accused of being witches were cruelly tortured and put to death largely in the Protestant countries. Sometimes self-appointed witch-hunters set out to hound down the guilty. In the orgy of witch-hunting thousands died dreadfully throughout Western Europe. The mentally deluded and the eccentric were caught up with the socially rebellious and the heretical. Many of those designated as witches were insane persons whose abnormal behaviour and utterances were seen as a threat to a settled society based on rigidly ordained beliefs and practices. They were, to a considerable extent, women, particularly elderly women whose mental aberrance or cantankerous nature was their only crime. An English chronicler wrote in 1584 'commonly they are doting, scolds, mad, divelish . . .'[15].

The extent to which Ireland became involved in the witch-craft delusion either before or after the Reformation was insignificant. The remoteness of the country reduced the impact of papal policies and continental practices on the early Irish Church and it tended to develop its own charac-teristics often to the chagrin of Rome. Apart from the Kyteler case there is no evidence of Catholic witch-burning in Ireland. The position did not change with the emergence of Protestantism even though it became an integral part of English government in Ireland. The failure of the Reformation to find roots among the native Irish meant that only the minority Protestant population was exposed to Protestant beliefs in the menace of witchcraft. Thus the pursuit of witches never really became an element of Irish society.

The one authenticated case of Irish witchburning took place in 1324 in Kilkenny. A wealthy local lady, Dame Alice le Kyteler, four times married, was accused by some of her children of having bewitched and killed their fathers. She was also said to have been involved in fortune telling and in trafficking in charms, magic powders and love philtres and in satanic rites, including sexual orgies. A solemn inquisition conducted by Richard Ledrede, Bishop of Ossory, accused her and ten associates, all from the ruling Anglo-Norman class, not only of *maleficia*, the satanic actions of a witch, but of heresy. It ended with one accomplice, Petronilla of Meath, being burnt publicly as a witch before a large con-course of people. Alice herself escaped a similar fate by fleeing to England, but a number of her other associates were tortured and burnt. It was the first time that the easy ways of the Irish Church had been disturbed by a trial for heresy. Some of the other Irish bishops, angered that Ledrede, a London Franciscan, should have initiated it, physically assaulted him at a subsequent meeting of bishops[16]. He fled to Avignon where he was able to persuade Pope Benedict XII, as well as the later Clement VI, that Ireland was full of demon-worshipping heretics but he later returned to his diocese ignoring the hostility of his fellow bishops[17].

Following the Reformation there is a record of two witches having been executed, also in Kilkenny, in 1578 on the direction of the lord-lieutenant, Sir William Drury. No details are extant about the witches or about the manner in which they were executed. It was reported that they were punished in accordance with 'natural law', as there was no statute law to sanction it, but this position was righted in 1586 when the Irish parliament enacted laws against witchcraft. The laws provided that for a first offence a witch would be imprisoned for one year and placed once in every quarter of the year in a public pillory for a period of six hours. For a second offence the punishment was death but there was no provision for torturing or burning alive at the stake[18].

Despite the legal provision there are few instances on record of subsequent witchcraft trials in Ireland. In 1661 Florence Newton of Youghal was accused of bewitching a servant girl and of the death of a man by kissing them. A trial took place; there is no record of the outcome but details of the evidence against the accused would suggest that she was mentally unstable[19]. The same was probably true of eight old women who were tried in Carrickfergus in 1711 for tormenting a young woman, Mary Dunbar, and causing her to have 'fits and ravings'. They were found guilty and, in accordance with law, imprisoned for twelve months and placed four times in a pillory. One of them had an eye beaten out while being stoned in the pillory[20]. This was the last such trial on record as having taken place in Ireland. Throughout Europe the witchcraft mania was now fast receding in the face of more enlightened and rational views. In Britain, where at least 30,000 persons had died at the stake during the previous two hundred years, parliament outlawed witchcraft in 1736; the Irish provisions, while not in use, were not repealed until 1829[21].

But there was a lingering folk belief in witches in some of the remoter parts of Ireland. In the Aran Islands, for instance, there was, towards the end of the last century, still some

21

credence in the *cailleach,* a hag capable of transferring mental illness from one person to another. An old woman who lived in Onaght on Inishmore was believed to possess such powers[22]. And, remarkably, in 1902, William Murphy, a cattle drover from Ballyporeen, Co. Tipperary, was charged before the local petty sessions with performing 'witchcraft' on his neighbours' cows at the dawn of a May morning. Although it is not clear what the statutory authority was, he was found guilty and sentenced to three months in Clonmel gaol[23].

These late instances of so-called witchcraft in remote areas of Ireland can hardly be linked to medieval heresy or the persecution of the insane. They were almost certainly the vestiges of a folklore rooted in the myths of pagan times. There is little doubt that they were a more valid reflection than the Kyteler case of the nature of Irish belief in witches.

Incarceration and Degradation

It can hardly be said that the onset of the Enlightenment, that period of the flowering of new ideas and attitudes during the later 17th century and the 18th century, brought with it a more understanding approach towards the insane. In some countries it may have ended their barbaric treatment as witches but it also led to a period extending to the nineteenth century marked by their inhuman and brutal treatment in prisons or other places of detention.

Ireland had avoided the earlier excesses of the rest of Europe because its traditional culture had remained largely intact owing to its remoteness and to the failure of the English administration to impose its authority to any notable degree. This had changed by the end of the seventeenth century. The violence of English armies, the systematic confiscation and settlement of Irish land, the application of harsh laws aimed at extirpating Irish Catholicism, had not only established absolute English control but had virtually destroyed the whole framework of Gaelic civilisation. From now on public measures, rare though they might be in regard to such social matters as provisions for the insane, would be English in origin and largely Protestant in inspiration.

The Protestant ethic placed great emphasis on an ordered society and on the obligation falling on the individual to behave and to conform. Drunkenness, vagrancy, blasphemy, witchcraft, all tended to disturb the religious and social order and demanded punishment. Insanity fell into the same

23

category since reason provided the norm and any deviation from it was a rejection by the individual of acceptable social standards. Irrationality was seen as a matter of deliberate and perverse choice rather than the inescapable consequence of an ill mind. In order to help maintain social conformity a public policy developed of incarcerating the non-conforming and the nuisance as well as the criminal. Little distinction was drawn between them. The beggar, the prostitute, the cripple, the scrofulous, the runaway apprentice, the imbecile and the mad were locked up in a variety of penal institutions where all were treated with great harshness.

As far as the insane were concerned there was nothing in this approach with which the dominant medical opinions of the period would disagree. Robert Burton in *The Anatomy of Melancholy* published in 1676 expresses contemporary views of the origins and treatment of insanity. Burton was a clergyman but his ideas were acceptable to his medical contemporaries. It was said that he had written the book with a view to relieving his own melancholy but that in the process it had increased to such a degree that nothing could make him laugh but the ribaldry of bargemen[1].

Burton's views were deeply rooted in the religious and superstitious beliefs of centuries with a gloss of Hippocratic medicine; they were to prevail until the beginning of the nineteenth century. According to them the basic source of madness was the Fall of Man and his consequent sinful nature. 'We are ... bad by nature, bad by kind but far worse by art, every man the greatest enemy unto himself' wrote Burton, but he recognised that there were some contributory causes such as bad air, the retention of bodily wastes and emotional disturbances[2].

In keeping with these views medical opinion sanctioned the incarceration and fettering of lunatics. It was in itself seen as an appropriate form of treatment even in the asylums established specifically for the insane. To confinement was frequently added a deliberate regimen of terrorisation. As late as 1812 Dunstan, the superintendent of St Luke's Hospital London, wrote, 'I consider fear the most effective principle by which to reduce the insane to orderly conduct'. In most of the principal European asylums until well into the nineteenth century the insane were subjected to copious blood-letting, starvation, flogging and terror in various forms[3].

No distinctions were made even if the patient was of considerable social standing. When in 1788 the British monarch George III developed what was believed to be insanity (modern medical opinion considers it to have been a rare metabolic disorder) his medical treatment described in a report circulated to members of the Irish parliament included 'coercion', a term implying shackling, beating and threatening with violent language. The report said that he had also been refused permission to read *King Lear* on the grounds that it was 'improper'[4].

A favoured method of inducing fear involved the threat of drowning. It was generally referred to as 'the bath of surprise' since it usually involved the sudden precipitation of the patient into deep water. He was sometimes thrown from a bridge into running water and caught with a net. A variation involved a practice somewhat similar to the buccaneer's method of keelhauling prisoners by tying the patient with a rope and dragging him through a river. According to Logan a somewhat similar practice was in use in Kerry about the end of the last century[5]. A more ingenious and terrifying method was used in some asylums. The patient was forced into a dark chamber one half of which consisted of an enormous cistern of water into which he inevitably fell while seeking an exit[6]. John Wesley, too, believed in terrorisation for 'raving madness'; he wrote, 'set the patient with his head under a great waterfall as long as his strength will bear'[7]. It appears that the essence of these treatments was to as nearly as possible kill the patient without exactly doing so.

Dr Achmet, otherwise known as Patrick Joyce or Patrick Kearns, who operated the Royal Patent Baths at Bachelors Walk, Dublin in the 1770s, used gentler methods of treatment by water. He claimed to cure successfully a multiplicity of disorders, including mental conditions, in hot and cold baths impregnated with such additions as putrifying horse manure. One lady who came to him with nerves in 'a deplorable state' found that, after a three-week course, they had become 'firm and restored to their natural tone, and her whole frame changed beyond her most sanguine hopes, for the better'[8].

Irish peasants had their own way of inducing terror, according to an account given by Lady Wilde. The patient was buried in a deep pit for three days and three nights with only his head left uncovered. During that period he was left without food; no communication with him was permitted. If he survived his living burial he was taken out more dead than alive and usually madder than ever but it was claimed that sometimes the madness had been frightened out of him[9].

The insane in jails

When during the seventeenth century the pressure began to develop for the institutional care of the more violently insane there was little public provision of any sort for the poor or the sick in Ireland. The monasteries had been closed. Here and there throughout the country there were small institutions like the Hospital of the Holy Trinity in New Ross founded by a local merchant and incorporated by a warrant of Queen Elizabeth; and the Hospital of the Holy Ghost in Waterford granted a charter by Henry VIII[10]. But they were few and of little significance. The Elizabethan poor law system had not been extended to Ireland. An unsympathetic Irish parliament enacted a number of provisions relating to the poor and homeless that were punitive in character, aimed at abating the nuisance of vagrancy rather than ameliorating the conditions of the lower orders. An Act of 1634 provided for the establishment of houses of correction in each county in which 'rogues' were to be confined[11]. They included:

- persons calling themselves scholars going about begging
- idle persons going about begging or using subtle craft
- fortune tellers
- persons being, or uttering themselves to be, collectors for jails
- fencers, bearwards and minstrels

- jugglers
- labourers able but refusing to work at reasonable wages
- persons delivered out of jail that beg for their fees or that otherwise travel begging
- pretenders to loss by fire
- gypsies.

Another Act of the same session of parliament added to the list of vagrants already subject to imprisonment those who were 'cosherers and wanderers' intimidating persons into giving lodging and food by threats 'of some scandalous rhyme or song'[12].

The houses of correction which subsequently developed, together with the jails, became not only the repositories of those specifically provided for by law but of others, including insane persons, who were a social nuisance or a threat to good order. Since the keepers and jailers were usually not paid by the State but depended on whatever fees they could extract from the prisoners and their relatives, the insane, usually moneyless and unwanted, were among the most disadvantaged. In 1684 the keeper of the Dublin House of Correction asked the City Assembly for some help towards maintaining 'madd women' and was given three pounds to cover a three month period. In 1701 the keeper was still looking for support for lunatics in his custody and on this occasion was granted two shillings weekly from the city revenue for each such person cared for by him. There was subsequently some minor provisions specifically for lunatics in Dublin. A number of cells were provided for them in the workhouse at James's Gate in 1708 largely on the initiative of the then lord mayor, Sir William Fownes. Some years later special provisions for insane soldiers were made in the Royal Hospital, Kilmainham when Sir Patrick Dun was physician there and they remained in existence, exclusively for military use, until 1849. But for most of the eighteenth century the jails, with a few minor exceptions, were the only centres in which lunatics could be confined[13].

The fact that those in charge of the various places of detention were unpaid and had almost total liberty in regard to the treatment of their prisoners made abuses inevitable. In 1729 a committee of the Irish House of Commons was told that John Hawkins, who was in charge of the main Dublin jails, Newgate and the Sheriff's Marshalsea, was treating many prisoners 'with the utmost cruelty and barbarity'. Rooms were rented to those who could pay for them; those unable to pay were locked in a dark, damp, underground dungeon. Sometimes male prisoners were thrown into 'the nunnery', the area in which 'strolling-women' were kept. Hawkins also carried on a considerable trade in the sale of liquor to the prisoners and those refusing to buy it were stripped and violently beaten. Some prisoners had not been committed by a magistrate but had been arbitrarily and unlawfully seized by Hawkins and incarcerated in chains until he could extort money for their release. In the light of the report the House of Commons decided to punish the keeper and a number of his subordinates and to bring in legislation to give better control over jails and jailers[14].

The small provision for lunatics made in the Dublin Workhouse in 1708 had increased to about forty places by 1729 when a new governing body was established to operate the institution largely as a foundling hospital[15]. The new governors decided to stop the admission of lunatics but it is clear from subsequent government reports that some provision continued to be made for them in the foulest of conditions.

The accommodation consisted of underground cells with unglazed windows where the inmates were chained in a state of indescribable misery. It was said that any inmates who subsequently recovered their senses had by then lost the use of their limbs because of the manacles and cramped space. Sometimes, for punishment, young children from the foundling hospital were incarcerated with them. Witnesses giving evidence to a parliamentary committee in 1758 recounted various horrors: a blind child locked up with a woman who was 'melancholy mad'; a blind madwoman, given to 'cursing and swearing', killed by a kick in the stomach from an official of the workhouse whom she had offended[16].

Since the cell accommodation was very limited the work-house did not free the Dublin jails of the insane where they continued to languish in conditions that became grimmer as the eighteenth century progressed. While occasional reforming measures were introduced they were little more than empty gestures. Two Acts of 1763 were concerned mainly with checking the extortions of the jailers and with improving the conditions of prisoners by such measures as providing for exercise grounds and separating the insane from the others[17]. Protestant clergymen were given authority to visit their local jails and to ensure that the prisoners had adequate food and medicine. In 1776 Dean Bayley made a public appeal for funds to enable the lunatics in the Bridewell to be fed and generally cared for and received a substantial contribution from John Rogerson of Carlow. But the general failure of the reforming laws was reflected in the various official reports of subsequent years. The fact was that the Irish parliament and the executive branches of government, exclusively Ascendancy in composition, were notoriously indifferent to the pursuit of social abuses in a largely disaffected population. Sixty years after the revealing report of 1729, John Howard, the Quaker reformer, visited the same jails and found a far more dreadful scene. In the Marshalsea prison some rooms were gin shops, whiskey was sold freely, 'reputed' wives were admitted and drinking and fighting went on continuously. Sometime earlier in the House of Lords, Lord Carysfort had described how in the same prison those able to pay the price could rent from their jailers a number of spare rooms which, he alleged, they filled with an assortment of dogs, pigs, fowls and whores. Howard also visited Newgate where prisoners lay dead and dying from intoxication or violence. As he passed through the prison on his tour of inspection he was robbed of his money and his gold watch[18].

During the 1780s considerable attention was given by parliamentary committees to Irish jail conditions. While pressure for reform was generated by a number of reports prepared by Howard the main impetus came from Jeremiah

Fitzpatrick, later knighted, a Dublin physician, who persistently confronted the government with the squalor and degradation of the existing system. He was particularly repelled by the mixture of the sane and the insane; in the Bridewell in James's Street, Dublin, young boys undergoing hard labour were locked with lunatics. In the same prison he noted 'supposedly insane women', some clearly not insane; one of those who appeared to be rational had been there for nine years. As a doctor he was in dread that the dungeons would become a breeding ground for epidemic disease and he feared that they would in time 'emit their noxious vapours to the destruction not only of the inhabitants of the jails but those of the city in general'[19].

Physical as well as mental disability could be a sufficient justification for confinement. Sir John Blacquiere, also campaigning for reform and one of the few socially concerned members of the Irish parliament, noted on a visit to the same jail that among the wretched objects of misery was:

> a young creature, about sixteen years old, of extraordinary beauty, who seemingly looked well and being asked why she did not move was answered by a man near her that if she did it was believed that her limbs, by the neglect and inveteracy of the disease, would break or fall in pieces under her[20].

The campaign led to a number of legislative measures; the most important innovation was the appointment of an inspector-general of prisons under an Act of 1786. Fitzpatrick had aired such a proposal in a pamphlet published two years earlier. Appropriately the lord-lieutenant now appointed him the first inspector-general[21].

Within a year there was ample evidence of deficiencies in the Act of 1786. Blacquiere and other reformers found little improvement in the lamentable conditions in the Dublin jails and, in an atmosphere of considerable sympathy for further reforms, new legislation, the Prisons Amendment Act of 1787 was enacted[22]. It strengthened the powers of the inspector-general and, where the insane were concerned, increased his authority by giving him the right to visit all public and private madhouses as often as he thought fit. Penalties were provided in the event of proprietors or keepers impeding such visits. But by the end of 1793 Fitzpatrick had turned his reforming zeal in another direction. He now applied himself to the problems of army health, particularly to soldiers' diet and their transport by sea, and leaving Ireland he passed from civilian to army employment[23].

Fitzpatrick's efforts had undoubtedly succeeded in removing some of the worst abuses and defaults in the prison system, particularly those perpetrated by the jailers themselves, but he had left his post as inspector-general before they were consolidated. Almost three years were to pass before his successor Rev Foster Archer was appointed. McDonagh has described him as 'a commonplace untrained and unenthusiastic functionary apparently appointed for political convenience and without any prior knowledge of, or interest in, the gaols'[24]. His reports towards the end of the 1790s show that the prisons were still wretched institutions and this continued to be the position over the next thirty years. The more favourable atmosphere for reform that existed in the 1780s had disappeared. Following the unsuccessful insurrection of 1798 there was no longer sympathy among those in authority for a prison population that now consisted to a large extent of the defeated and the subversive; a disaffected element contaminated by ideas about political liberty and the rights of man. The fact that Dr Trevor, medical officer to Kilmainham Jail, felt in 1808 that he could fill the post of inspector-general more effectively than Archer is an indication of how some of those then involved with the prison system perceived the desirable qualities for that office. Trevor, who had held his prison appointment since 1798 wrote, on the basis of a previous promise, to a government official pressing that Archer's job be given to him[25]. He added:

> I need not, I think, observe to you that from my exertions I am particularly obnoxious to the dis-

affected of this country and it was under that consideration the promise was made as in case any
accident should happen to me my family would be
left ill provided for . . .

His own assessment of himself was in accord with what
others thought of him. During the same year Richard Brinsley
Sheridan calling for a parliamentary investigation into Irish
jails described Trevor as 'of the most inhuman, hardened and
malignant disposition'. His request for the inspector-general
post was not granted and the prison population was left to
the mercy of Archer's apathy rather than Trevor's malig-
nancy[26].

Throughout the early years of the nineteenth century the
conditions in the prisons were as bad as they had ever been.
The insane were being imprisoned both as criminals and as
debtors without any special provision for them. Disorder and
oppression prevailed. Turnkeys were given free rein to extract
'garnish' from the unfortunate inmates; in the Four Courts
Marshalsea, a debtor's prison, a bed cost seven shillings and
seven pence a week; five pence secured a bundle of straw;
the moneyless lay on the hard flagstones. There were no lights
during the hours of darkness; a prisoner wrote 'the most
shocking wickedness is committed by men and women at
night'. To the din of the intoxicated and the mad was added
the noise of dogs; the same prisoner wrote 'they bark and
fight day and night; they puke and shit on the stairs and in
the passages and make quarrels between their owners and
other prisoners[27].

An indication of the official attitude of the period towards
the prisons can be seen in the site selected for a jail in Cork.
It was subject to extensive flooding. When the mayor of the
city pointed it out as a matter of interest to Sir Arthur
Wellesley (later Duke of Wellington) who was on a visit to
the city in 1807 the latter was reported as having remarked
sarcastically: 'I suppose this is being done from motives of
economy to save the hangman's fee, for if you do not choose
to hang them you may drown them'. Subsequently another

was chosen[28].

During the 1820s the most wretched conditions of all appear to have existed in the county bridewells which, for most of the country, were the only local centres in which lunatics could be detained. The inspectors' report for 1823 describes them graphically:

> They are wretched places of confinement one of which is to be found in each town and village. . . . In a miserable building prisoners are confined for days and weeks, without yards for exercise, without inspection, care of health or morals; men and woman are thrown together in cold cells without bedding, on damp clay floors. No chaplain attends; no surgeon or physician is appointed; no regular supply of food is provided; all is fraud, oppression and misery.

One of the inspectors described Youghal Bridewell as 'the worst regulated prison I have ever visited'. A prisoner who had been confined there for three years was permitted to operate in his cell what was euphemistically described as a 'musical academy'. It was a 'scene of shameful disorder and dissipation' to which visitors were freely admitted to participate in the revels[29].

Two well-known English Quakers, Elizabeth Fry and her brother John, who visited most of the Irish jails in 1827 found a similar picture[30]. They were particularly critical of the conditions of the lunatics and the lack of attention to them. Many lay on bundles of straw in solitary confinement in a 'very offensive state'; some were mixed with other prisoners. In a few instances old jail buildings had been set aside exclusively for the insane; in Lifford they were 'kindly treated' but in Roscommon their condition was 'pitiful in the greatest degree'. Another visitor to the Roscommon building five years later saw female lunatics with iron clasps around their bodies fastened with chains to the walls and other patients sitting 'like wild beasts' in cages of iron[31].

The lord-lieutenant, Wellesley, had replaced Archer as inspector-general in 1822 by two appointees, Major James

Palmer and Major Benjamin Woodward. The creation of a second post had probably more to do with the appointment of both a Catholic and a Protestant than with a desire to improve conditions in the prisons. The government, placating Catholic opinion by gradually removing former restrictions and disabilities, was particularly anxious to demonstrate the absence of religious bias in public institutions which, in the past, were often centres of proselytism. There is no evidence that the two new inspectors were any more effective than Archer had been. Palmer, in particular, could hardly have commanded much authority or influence since he himself underwent a period of imprisonment as a debtor in Kilmainham Jail during his period of office. The fact that he continued to hold his post then, and subsequently, was in itself an indication of the government's general indifference towards prison reform[32].

The houses of industry

By the end of the eighteenth century the jails had been supplemented by the houses of industry. They were established by a statute of 1772 following a campaign conducted by Dr Richard Woodward, Dean of Clogher, seeking measures to relieve the public of the nuisance of proliferating beggars particularly in the cities and towns[33].

The Act was punitive rather than charitable in design. Its harsh provisions were intended to suppress 'undeserving' beggars by forcibly committing them to the houses of industry where they could be detained for up to four years. The 'deserving' poor were to be given a badge permitting them to beg so that they would remain dependent on private charity and not on public funds. The infirm poor were, however, to be admitted voluntarily to the institutions. The Act made no reference to the insane and it was generally understood that they were to be admitted only in exceptional circumstances. In time, however, they came to form a large segment of the inmates.

The government's intention was that every county should provide a house of industry for its own poor. However, the local grand juries with whom the initiative lay were largely indifferent and only a small number of institutions was established notably those in Dublin, Cork, Waterford, Limerick and Clonmel. In the circumstances Dublin continued to bear the brunt of providing for the Irish beggar population, many of whom flocked to it from all over the country. While there was no legislative sanction for it, the Dublin House of Industry, based on an old malt-house in Chanel Row, assumed the character of a national establishment and received special financial support as such from the government[34]. It quickly became a centre reflecting the whole spectrum of human wretchedness in Ireland. Although life within its walls may have been better than in jail the gallimaufry of the hungry, the homeless, the diseased and the outcast of all ages made unavoidable a scene of squalor and hopelessness.

The governors, who had initially adopted a policy of admitting the insane for short periods only when they were without any means whatever, soon found themselves under pressure to provide special accommodation. Reports and correspondence of the period show the governors in a favourable light and genuinely concerned about the general lack of provision for the insane. Ten cells were provided in the house in 1776 and two years later these and other accommodation in the institution were housing forty-five lunatics some of whom had been transferred from the dreadful conditions of the bridewell in James's Street. Twenty of them were employed on menial duties in the house at a weekly wage of two pence each. Under growing pressure the governors increased the number of cells and by 1808 appear to have had special provision for seventy-six lunatics all of whom were 'maniacs (requiring) confinement and coercion' but there were many others accommodated with physically ill persons in wards where, in general, there were 'more than two persons to each bed'. Understandably a visitor to the institution at this time described it as a 'scene of dirt, of noise, of confusion, of madness, of everything that was abominable'[35].

Conditions for the insane in some of the other houses of

industry during the early years of the nineteenth century were no better. In Clonmel where thirty-six cells were provided in 1811 they lay naked in a yard on bundles of straw and those in the vicinity could hear their 'bellowing and hideous noise'. In 1814 Henry Sergent, mayor of Waterford, writing to the chief secretary said that the local house of industry had inadequate funds to give the insane proper care[36].

In Limerick Edward Smyth, a local doctor, built at his own expense a small asylum for lunatics adjoining the house of industry. Its operation was taken over by the governors who soon found themselves unable to finance both institutions, and the mayor, Thomas Wilkinson, reported to the chief secretary during 1814 that a number of local citizens had to be asked to subscribe 'to keep the wretched inmates from being let loose on the community'. Thomas Spring Rice, a local landlord, gave a graphic picture to a parliamentary committee in 1817 of conditions in this house of industry. He was one of its governors and over the next twenty years was to be a major influence on the reform of Irish provisions for the insane. The Limerick accommodation consisted of an open arcade behind which stone-floored cells had been constructed. There was no heating and the patients sometimes died when exposed to the extremities of the weather. Two, and on occasions three, patients occupied each cell of about six feet by ten feet. Those in a state of 'furious insanity' were restrained by having their hands passed under their knees and manacled in that position. Their ankles were secured with bolts. Because of the length of confinement in that posture some lost the power of their limbs and became no longer capable of rising. The less agitated lunatics were confined with physically sick inmates in rooms over the cells where dead and dying sometimes lay together. Rice saw in one of the rooms a woman seated with the corpse of a child on her knees; the child had been dead for two days and was almost 'in a state of putridity'. The 'most atrocious profligacy' prevailed and the keeper of the lunatics, who was later dismissed, claimed exclusive sexual rights to the females in his care. An English visitor had, a few years earlier, described similar scenes there. They included 'a raving maniac . . . handcuffed to a stone of 300 pounds weight which, with the most horrible yells, by a convulsive effort of strength, he dragged from one end of the room to the other'. Yet according to the visitor, John Carr, the governor appeared to be a humane man who 'seemed deeply to regret what he could not conceal'[37].

Lunatics at large

One of the reasons for the increasing pressure for the admission of lunatics to the houses of industry, particularly the Dublin institution, was the growing demand to confine the many disturbed and uncontrolled persons who were wandering abroad. For centuries, in the absence of institutions, they had been tolerated; now that tolerance was fading as the system of jails and houses of industry offered the possibility of controlling them.

The Marquis de Latocnaye after a visit to Ireland in 1796-7 commented: 'one of the most painful spectacles to be seen in nearly all the principal towns of Ireland is the number of weak-minded persons in the streets'[38]. Another visitor, Edward Wakefield, told a parliamentary committee in 1815 that on journeys throughout the country he had seen pauper maniacs who were 'the sport of the common people' and the same committee later reported that lunatics were allowed to wander until those who were 'outrageous' were taken up and sent to Dublin[39]. Two years later a reforming English politician, George Rose, claimed during a parliamentary debate that in Ireland idiots were the subject of 'public sport' and that 'unruly maniacs were suffered to go about the country the terror of the neighbourhood in which they resided'[40]. Crofton Croker, an English visitor, wrote in 1824 that insane persons were to be found wandering on most roads and that some had acquired vicious habits notably 'throwing stones which they do with great dexterity'. He complained that for years one particular idiot had been tolerated on the road from Cork to Carrigaline where he was given 'to pinching unprotected women on the back and arms'[41]. A local clergyman claimed that in the Armagh area about this time the sight of the many homeless lunatics was 'a grievous and affecting spectacle'[42].

Some families who had severely physically or mentally disabled members exhibited them in public places with the hope of provoking sympathy and receiving alms. They gathered outside churches and at fairs and holy wells. An indignant correspondent in the *Cork Advertiser* in 1816, urging institutional provision for them, wrote that 'the most shocking objects are exhibited . . . their exposure is often attended with the most fatal consequences to delicate females in the state of pregnancy'[43].

Not all lunatics were allowed to wander abroad or placed on public display. Sometimes in rural Ireland an insane person was confined in his own home if his family wished him to avoid becoming the butt of public amusement or an inmate of some wretched place of detention. But the impoverished cabin home of the typical peasant family allowed for only the most primitive of provisions. The practice was to dig a pit either in the floor of the cabin or in an outhouse and to confine the patient in it. The pit was covered by a crib, a lattice of stout rods; it was relatively shallow so that the patient could not stand up and was more easily controllable. This became his permanent abode; here he was fed and lived until he died. Where circumstances permitted there were variations in his manner of home care. An account of a case in County Limerick in about 1820 described how the insane wife of a farmer was kept in the vault of a ruined castle tied by a chain to a heavy harrow. She succeeded in escaping and climbed ninety feet to the top of the chimney of the ruin where she remained for a period to 'the astonishment and terror of the spectators'[44].

Before the coming of the asylums insanity in the peasant family was usually accepted stoically as a cross it had to bear; there was no one to turn to for advice; no hope of cure unless they believed in the miraculous powers of Glannagalt or one of the other places of pilgrimage already described. Sometimes they were taken advantage of by the mountebanks who flourished in a simple unsophisticated society. Quacks 'with the cure' whose assistance had been called upon sometimes belaboured a demented person with a hawthorn stick while uttering gibberish interspersed with Latin words and dashing holy water on the patient and his surroundings. Eventually they would announce that the devil had gone out of the patient; occasionally they would acknowledge defeat. In either event they would have been rewarded for their intervention by copious amounts of whiskey consumed during the exorcistic ritual.

Lady Wilde has described a case of quackery that appears to have occurred about the beginning of the nineteenth century[45]. Davy Flynn from Roscommon became suddenly mad and the local quack was called. He declared that the lunatic was not Davy Flynn but was an old charger belonging to a French general who had come to Ireland at the time of the insurrection. The real Davy was in fairyland and his substitute would have to be well fed with food suitable for a horse. His friends thereupon rammed oats and straw down the throat of the unfortunate maniac who, eventually breaking loose, pursued them with hideous yells and curses. Finally he was tied down and incarcerated locally where he eventually died to the relief of his friends who continued to believe that he had been transformed into a French charger. It is difficult not to regard the story as apocryphal.

Transport to Dublin

The growing demands for the control of the more unruly and dangerous of those permitted to wander at large and the lack of local provision for them led to an attempt by the government in an Act of 1787 to establish a county system of special wards[46]. While the legislation was not very specific it implied that the wards should be associated with county infirmaries by assigning accountability to the surgeons of these institutions for any public funds spent on the measures. As the infirmaries, the only public facilities statutorily provided for sick people, were already being grossly neglected by the grand juries responsible for their supervision, the new legislation was almost entirely ignored. Thirty years later there was not a single cell for the insane in twenty-four counties[47]. In the circumstances if a place could not be found in the local jail the lunatic had to be transported to a house of industry willing to take him. As these were few in number the Dublin house of industry with its national obligations offered to most parts of the country the only possibility of help.

One difficulty was that there was no clear legal provision for raising the costs of transport. Richard Edgeworth, father of the novelist Maria, had written in 1808 to Sir Andrew Halliday of Manchester, an influential campaigner for better provisions for the insane in Britain and Ireland, drawing attention to Irish conditions and suggesting that it was essential to empower magistrates to raise funds 'to transmit wandering idiots and madmen to Dublin'[48]. However no changes were made in the law; most grand juries appeared to be able to raise the necessary funds without difficulty, probably finding sufficient sanction for doing so in the Act of 1787[49].

Patients were taken from many parts of the country on what was frequently a long and wretched journey over the rough roads of the period. In 1815 the houses of industry in Cork, Waterford, Limerick, Ennis, Clonmel and Kilkenny all had lunatics from outside their areas. Nearly one third of those in Waterford were from distant parts of the country. But the majority of those who sought accommodation outside their own areas were taken to Dublin, some from remote parts of the West and North, in a manner described by a parliamentary committee as 'shocking to humanity'[50].

The practice was to tie them with a rope to the back of a cart and to force them to walk behind it to Dublin no matter the distance. The parliamentary enquiry was told that since the rope was normally attached tightly to the lunatics' wrists 'mortification' was often produced and that at least one in every five of the patients had subsequently to have an arm amputated[51]. Denis Browne, MP for Mayo, told another enquiry in 1817 that incurable lunatics from Mayo were sent to Dublin at two guineas each in the care of carriers who treated them 'very brutally'. In the Dublin house of industry

he had enquired about thirty or forty patients sent previously from Mayo but could trace only one woman. No
account of the others could be given to him, whether they
had died, or were cured or had ever arrived there[52]. This was
not surprising. Robert Peel, the chief secretary in Ireland who
had been responsible for initiating the enquiry to which
Browne contributed, had earlier told the House of Commons
that it was 'common practice' for carriers to leave insane
persons 'in the most deplorable state' outside the door of the
house of industry without waiting to find out whether they
could be accepted[53].

The method of conveying patients to distant centres was but
one of an accumulation of cruelties associated with the treatment of the insane which eventually served to hasten a new
era of care. In an age becoming more sensitive to human
rights the so-called enlightenment that sanctioned cruelty
was slowly giving way to a new rationality that rejected the
view that the mistreatment of the insane could be justified.

Fools, Mad and Jonathan Swift

In one way or another Jonathan Swift, the illustrious founder of Ireland's first hospital for the insane, lived with madness all his life. Born after the death of his father he became closely dependent, particularly for his education, on the assistance of a paternal uncle, Godwin. Godwin died insane in 1688[1]. His uncle's insanity probably marked the young Swift's introduction to the reality of madness, a condition that continued to interest him until he died, ironically and mistakenly, a certified lunatic himself. It was a subject that provided material for his barbed pen; one that, in his view, clearly had relevancy to the contemporary politicians, churchmen and others whose foibles and posturings caused him continuing indignation.

It figured in one of his earliest and most famous satires, *A Tale of a Tub* published in 1704[2]. This allegorical story provides a vehicle for acerbic comment on the main Christian churches as well as containing a number of lengthy digressions, including one on the condition of madness which clearly reflects the view of the times that equated lunacy with moral weakness. In it Swift suggests that madness is the origin of all great historical events and changes. The sane person, living a serene life, is happy to continue in that condition and is unlikely to think about subduing multitudes to his own power or vision. All great revolutions whether in politics, philosophy, or religion have had their origin in mad minds.

Swift puts forward ironically the proposition that insane

42

persons could be made useful citizens if they were assigned
roles in keeping with their behaviour. He described one type
of incarcerated lunatic as

> ... tearing his straw in piecemeal, swearing and blas-
> pheming, biting his grate, foaming at the mouth and
> emptying his pisspot in the spectators faces.

Here Swift sees the makings of an ideal army officer; such a
patient should, he suggests, be put in command of a regiment
and sent into battle. On the other hand the 'eternally talking'
lunatic would make a good parliamentarian while the grovelling
patient, gabbling meaningless compliments, would make an
accomplished royal courtier because of his capacity for
flattery.

In 1714, ten years after the publication of *A Tale of a Tub*,
Swift became a governor of Bedlam (Bethlehem) Hospital in
London where he had gone to from Dublin to take up an appointment. There is no record that he ever attended a meeting.
Bedlam was probably the most notorious of all institutions
for the insane at that period; the public paid to view and
taunt the lunatics in their cages and although nominally a
hospital it appeared to lack any degree of humanity. It seemed
a fit object for the *saeva indignatio*, the savage indignation
of Swift's self-written epitaph, but there is no indication that
it was then aroused. On the contrary, there is evidence from
Swift's own correspondence with his friend Stella that he,
too, had viewed Bedlam as a place of entertainment. Some
years before he had become a governor he had gone one day
on an outing with a party of friends that included women
and children. Starting at the Tower, where they watched the
lions, they went on to see the horrors of Bedlam whence they
progressed to a chop-house, eventually ending what appeared
to be an enjoyable day at a puppet-show[3].

Although Swift left London and returned to Dublin within
six months of his appointment as a governor of Bedlam he
continued to retain that office. He apparently regarded the
hospital as good enough for the care of his friends. During
1722 he wrote to its secretary arranging the admission of an

insane friend, Jo Beaumont, who had taken to galloping on horseback through the streets of London throwing his money to the rabble. Beaumont, a mathematically inclined linen-draper from Trim, was believed to have gone mad from thinking too long about the intricacies of calculating longitude[4].

Swift's apparent acceptance of conditions in Bedlam was a reflection of the prevailing view that saw no place for kindness, compassion or comfort in the treatment of the insane. When later he turned his attention to the need for a lunatic asylum in Dublin his primary motivation appears to have been that there should be a special institution to house the insane and allow them to be removed from the jails and the streets rather than that there should be a hospital based on a more humane regimen. Swift's own perception of what conditions in his hospital were likely to be can be seen in one of his last and bitterest poems, *A Character, Panegyric and Description of the Legion Club*, written in 1736[5]. Here he venomously attacks the members of the Irish parliament for whom he visualises special cells in his proposed madhouse:

> While they sit a picking straws
> Let them rave of making laws
> While they never hold their tongue
> Let them dabble in their dung.

And referring to two particular members he urges:

> Tie them, keeper, in a tether
> Let them stare and stink together
> Both are apt to be unruly
> Lash them daily, lash them duly.

This is, of course, the exaggerated language of satire but the vision it conjures up of the then treatment of the insane is accurate and there is no indication in this poem or elsewhere that Swift found it reprehensible or in need of reformation. While he was intolerant and egocentric, he was a compassionate man whose rages often arose from his concern about the down-trodden. The *Modest Proposal*, probably his most scathing satirical pamphlet, was an outburst of indignation at the miseries to which Irish pauper children were being subjected; yet remarkably for the founder of one of the first asylums for the insane one finds no evidence of sympathy for them in his works. In that regard he was simply a man of his times.

The Dean's hospital

The first move to provide a hospital for the insane in Dublin came as early as 1699 when an anonymous donor offered to the city corporation through an intermediary, Dr Thomas Molyneaux, subsequently state physician, a sum of £2,000 towards the cost of maintaining a hospital for aged lunatics and diseased persons. The corporation initially accepted the offer and decided to give £200 towards the building costs on a site which the Earl of Athlone had donated within St James's Gate. The task of raising the additional sum necessary to build the hospital was left to 'well disposed citizens'[6]. It does not appear that there were many of them but, in any event, probably because of the hordes of beggars in the city streets, the corporation later decided to reallocate the site for the Dublin Workhouse which opened in 1703. The main purpose of the workhouse, to which reference has already been made, was to reduce the nuisance of beggars, a somewhat forlorn hope in view of their numbers and general lawlessness[7].

Some years after the opening of the workhouse, William Fownes, the then lord mayor and an *ex officio* governor of the workhouse, concerned at the lack of special provision for the insane, arranged to have added to it six cells for 'the most outrageous'. Fownes was unhappy about the lack of public institutions for the destitute and diseased in general. He was one of the city's patriarchs, a wealthy member of the Irish parliament with an estate in Wicklow, a villa adjoining the Phoenix Park and a town-house off College Green in the shadow of the parliament buildings where the city rabble tended to gather in large numbers[8]. By the 1720s it was evident that the workhouse in James's Street was fast becoming a repository for foundlings to the exclusion of others and was failing to make any real impact on the generality of the city's destitute.

In a pamphlet published in 1725 Fownes proposed that there should be further measures; 'deserving poor' should be confined to their own parish and allowed to beg within its boundaries; inveterate 'vagabonds and beggars' should be subjected to the harsh regime of a workhouse until they promised to give up begging[9]. These proposals failed to generate any action; in any event pamphlets on social and political issues proliferated at this period and were usually seen as little more than the literary flatulence of ambitious politicians and churchmen.

To the failure of his pamphlet was added the disappointment of a decision made in 1729 by the reconstituted governing body of the workhouse to stop the admission of insane persons[10]. By then about forty lunatics were housed there but since the workhouse had now taken on the character of a foundling hospital the new governors decided that it would have been incongruous if it were also to serve as a centre for the insane. As already mentioned, this policy did not prevent the retention in its cells of some mad persons one of whose uses was the terrorisation of children locked in with them when they broke the rules of the foundling hospital[11].

It is reasonable to assume that Swift was conscious of the decision of the governors of the workhouse to reject the insane when in November 1731 he announced his intention of providing in his will for the establishment of a lunatic asylum. This announcement was contained in the final quatrain of his cynical poem *Verses on the Death of Dr Swift*:

> He gave the little Wealth he had
> To build a House for Fools and Mad
> And shew'd by one satyric Touch
> No Nation wanted it so much[12].

Since he does not appear to have had any views of his own as to the requirements of a lunatic asylum he consulted Fownes, who was possibly the only public figure likely to have a special interest in the subject. Fownes himself had earlier given some thought to the need for a hospital of this sort. He had dismissed the idea on the grounds that it might

be overwhelmed by the demands for admission as well as
giving rise to the risk that it might lead to 'husbands and wives
trying who could first get the other to Bedlam' as, he believed,
was the English experience. But by now he had dropped his
reservations and, convinced that the complete lack of provision required urgent action, he wrote enthusiastically to
Swift in September, 1732, outlining his own ideas for a hospital
and urging the raising of public subscriptions with Swift's
support[13]. In his view the hospital should be located at a
distance from dwelling houses since the 'cries and exclamations
of the outrageous would reach a great way'. He had in mind
a piece of land belonging to St Patrick's Cathedral alongside
the almshouse for girls operated by Mary Mercer of which
'she is weary'. It was an open space at the bottom of what is
now South King Street and was popularly known as 'The
Dunghill'[14].

Fownes suggested a scheme for the layout of the hospital
based on London's Bedlam; this would enable the building to
be started quickly, without the need for plans or an architect.
It would be initially restricted to six or eight cells for the
'outrageous'. His proposals differed in a fundamental respect
from Swift's aims. Swift always appeared to have had in mind
a hospital for pauper lunatics, and this was borne out by his
later will, but Fownes envisaged a private madhouse where
friends and relations would pay for the support of the
lunatics.

Fownes's enthusiasm and anxiety to get a hospital established quickly appear to have been a deterrent rather than an
encouragement to Swift and there is no record of any response
from him to Fownes's proposals. Apart from the fact that
they appeared to differ over the aim of the hospital
it had never been Swift's intention that the hospital should
become a reality in his own lifetime. Since he had few funds
readily available at this time any hospital then built would
have had to depend largely on public subscription as Fownes
envisaged, and ran the risk of perpetuating the name of
Fownes as its founder rather than the egocentric Dean. Swift
stuck to his original intention that the establishment of the

hospital was an event that would follow his demise and that he would provide for it in his will.

But by 1735 he was becoming worried as to whether the hospital would become a reality even then. Since he was not a wealthy man his estate was likely to be relatively small and he could not be sure that other benefactors would be disposed to supplement it. The problem was not only that the plight of the insane attracted little public sympathy but that there were other charitable institutions developing which were more likely to attract the support of the philanthropically minded and the acclaim of the public. Hospitals for the pauper sick such as the Charitable Infirmary, Dr Steevens Hospital, Mercer's Hospital and the first maternity hospital in Ireland, the Rotunda Hospital, were coming into existence and all of them were seeking benefactors[15]. It appeared to Swift that if he were to acquire a site for it during his lifetime this would give a greater promise of the eventual opening of his own hospital.

The site suggested in Fownes's proposal was no longer available as it had been handed over by Mary Mercer for a new hospital which was to bear her own name. During 1735 he approached Dublin Corporation for a plot at Oxmantown Green. Writing then to the city recorder he lamented the fact that the lack of a public-spirited friend had left him unable to purchase a site himself and he criticised 'the neighbouring country squires always watching like crows over a carcase over every estate that was likely to be sold . . .'. The corporation agreed to let him have a plot of land at the nominal rent of a peppercorn annually. It was only then that the Dean's intention to found an asylum became generally known and a popular monthly magazine reflecting the esteem in which he was held, commented:

> The Dean must die our idiots to maintain!
> Perish ye idiots: and long live the Dean![16]

For reasons unknown the city council failed to honour its promise to give him a site. Swift's growing exasperation is evident from subsequent correspondence. 'I wish I had any certainty in the matter' (of the hospital becoming a reality) he wrote in 1737 to Robert Cope, a member of the Irish House of Commons, expressing fears that parliament might be contemplating legislation preventing legacies to public charities[17]. For a brief period he considered handing over the development of the asylum to the governors of Dr Steevens Hospital but dropped the idea following the death of a medical friend, Sir Richard Helsham, who was supporting it[18].

In July, 1738, he wrote sorrowfully to his publisher, George Faulkner, proprietor of *Faulkner's Journal*: 'I believe no man had ever more difficulty, or less encouragement, to bestow his whole fortune for a charitable use'[19]. He arranged for Faulkner to publish an advertisement informing the public that while Swift intended to leave his whole fortune to establish a hospital it was then all tied up in loans, land and other securities and he had insufficient ready funds with which to acquire a site. There is no evidence that this *cri de coeur* aroused any particular interest and by May 1740, when he eventually made his will, he had given up the quest for the acquisition of a site during his own lifetime.

By now Swift was in his early 70s and his health was deteriorating. In 1741 with his memory going he was deaf and beginning to act irrationally. He had a premonition that this would happen. Many years previously, looking at the withered upper branches of a great elm, he had remarked, 'I shall be like that tree; I shall die at the top'[20]. The modern medical interpretation of his symptoms indicates that he was probably suffering from senile decay aggravated by thrombophlebitis[21] but in the view of Swift's contemporaries he was a madman. It was a view compounded of ignorance and malice. His friend, Lord Orrery, describing his behaviour in 1742, wrote:

> His rage increased absolutely to the degree of madness; in this miserable state he seemed to be appointed as the first proper inhabitant of his own hospital especially as from an outrageous lunatic he sunk after-

wards into a quite speechless idiot . . .[22].

In accordance with the legal provisions of the period for the protection of the interests of insane persons with property, a process, *de lunatico inquirendo*, was carried out during 1742 by commissioners and a jury. They concurred in the view that he was 'a person of unsound mind and memory and not capable of taking care of his person'. The jury included a chandler, a brewer, two carpenters, a currier (dresser of tanned leather) and a hosier[23]. Swift's 'savage indignation' would have been put to the test if he had been aware that his mental state was being judged by such unlettered persons so far removed from the intellectual world in which he had been a lion for so long. But he was beyond knowing. He had run, ruminated Stephen Dadalus, 'to the wood of madness, his mane foaming in the moon, his eyeballs stars'[24]. He died, mentally isolated from the world around him, in 1745.

Swift died worth about £12,000 of which £11,000 was to be used for the hospital. His will provided for the purchase of lands in any province of Ireland except Connaught, the income from which would go towards the purchase of a site beside Dr Steevens Hospital on which an asylum would be built for the reception of as many 'idiots and lunatics' as the income from the land could support. It was to be called St Patrick's Hospital. Swift directed his executors to apply for a royal charter to incorporate the hospital and this was granted by George II in August 1746[25].

The majority of the original governors were friends of Swift; eight of the total of fourteen were clergymen including the Protestant primate and Swift's successor as Dean of St Patrick's. They acted quickly; Dr Steevens Hospital leased a site for an annual rental of £10 and George Semple, a Dublin architect, was chosen to plan the new institution. Building started in 1748 and with the assistance of additional benefactors including a legacy from Dr Stearne, Bishop of Clogher, wards endowed by Sir Richard Levinge and Alderman Ben Bower, and grants amounting to £2,000 from the Irish parliament the hospital was opened to the first patients in 1757[26]. While officially titled St Patrick's Hospital it was for a considerable period to be popularly known as Swift's Hospital.

From the beginning there was difficulty in funding it. Swift had not been particularly business-like; some of his creditors were devious and unreliable and the governors had considerable difficulty in gathering together his assets. A farmer named Denn from Saggart to whom Swift had lent £2,120 was discovered not to own the lands on which he had given a mortgage to the Dean. James Clinch of Newcastle who collected tithes to which Swift was entitled refused to account fully for all the monies and legal proceedings had to be taken against him to recover them. Mrs Brent, the Dean's housekeeper, and her daughter Mrs Ridgeway who operated a benevolent scheme devised and funded by Swift involving the giving of interest free loans of £5 to poor tradesmen were found to have kept their accounts in an 'irregular and confused' manner. Within six years of the opening of the hospital the governors faced with the reality that the annual income from Swift's estate was no more than £4,000 and capable of supporting only about fifty patients decided to petition parliament for support[27].

The Commons was well disposed towards the hospital and agreed to a grant of £1,000 for it in November 1763. Four years later it decided to provide continuing support for St Patrick's. By 1800, as a result of parliamentary grants and further legacies and donations, the hospital had been considerably extended and then accommodated 158 patients[28].

The first master of the hospital, William Drugden, was a relation of Swift and was appointed to his post while the hospital was still in planning. He died before it opened and was succeeded by Thomas Dyton who lived in the hospital and continued to carry on a printing business in Dame Street. In accordance with the general practice of the times St Patrick's continued under lay rather than medical management until 1858 when the first medical master, John Trench Gill, was appointed. There were, however, visiting physicians at all times including such distinguished personalities as

Robert Emmet (1770-1803), father of the patriot; James Cleghorn (1803-25); John Crampton (1825-40) and Charles Croker (1840-70)[29].

The earliest patients had to be accompanied on admission by a complete history of their illness certified by the minister and churchwardens of the parish from which they came. It was also necessary for security to be given that the patient would be taken back on discharge, for the payment of sixpence a week for washing and for the lodgement of twenty shillings to defray funeral expenses should the patient die while in hospital[30]. This latter provision was common to the hospitals of the period.

Faced with the difficulty of operating the hospital on a very restricted income the governors decided to admit paying patients or, as they were called, 'boarders' and by 1800 a third of all those in residence were paying for their care. During 1783 advertisements in the Dublin newspapers which had been drafted by Dr Emmet suggested that persons sending boarders to the hospital would not only be making a 'comfortable provision' for them but would also be performing an act of charity by helping to provide for 'poor fellow creatures' not in a position to contribute[31]. Emmet had become the great strength of the hospital after his appointment. He worked for some years without any remuneration other than that to which his public office of state physician entitled him, examining and certifying all patients admitted, acting as physician as well as keeping the accounts of the hospital. Eventually the governors decided that he should receive a sum of two guineas quarterly in respect of each boarder[32].

By the beginning of the nineteenth century the admission rules had been changed to reflect not only the social mixture of the patients but the increasing status of the medical profession. Boarders were admitted by the master on the certificate of a doctor. Pauper patients were also admitted on the basis of a medical certificate but only after consideration of their case by the board of governors. The fees for the boarders varied between 30 guineas and 100 guineas a year, those paying the maximum fee being allocated two rooms as well as a servant for their exclusive use. For a period boarders also had the privilege of access to a piano kept by the master in his private quarters. Since all paying patients were required to bring their own bedding to the hospital there was a great variety of it to be seen in the wards, ranging from large four-posted beds with tent roofs to much simpler provisions[33].

Most of the menial work of the hospital was carried out by the pauper patients who were not admitted to the company of the boarders except in a servile capacity. In keeping with the times the boarders appear to have had a sharp sense of their social superiority. According to a parliamentary report:

> . . . most of these unhappy persons have a most lively recollection of the rank in life to which they may still be considered to belong; the disease of many more develops itself on the assumption of one much higher[34].

The policy of having paying patients was quite contrary to the hospital's charter which had interpreted Swift's wishes as intending the hospital to be exclusively for the use of paupers. Nevertheless, this continued to be the practice until 1842 when Lord Chancellor Sugden drew attention to its illegality. All paying patients were then transferred to private institutions. In 1888 the governors had an amendment made to the hospital's charter legalising the taking of fees; the admission of paying patients was resumed and St Patrick's became and remained largely a private hospital[35].

Historically St Patrick's Hospital is of interest because it was not only Ireland's first hospital for the insane but the legacy of one of the great figures of the eighteenth century. While the patients during its early history were undoubtedly cared for in a more humane setting than if they had been confined in the jails and houses of industry of the period it was not a pioneering hospital and not in the forefront of the moral treatment movement described later. The hospital's regimen was a product of its times and not in advance of them. Coercion and restraint were general. Chairs had been built firmly into the walls in which difficult lunatics were secured with metal attachments. Little attention was paid to cleanliness and there was a belief that the patients were insensitive to cold[36]. The board minutes of the hospital would suggest that until the 1830s the governors showed little interest in hospital conditions or treatment and concerned themselves mainly with financial matters, the admission of patients and the appointment of staff. As late as 1835 the commissioners enquiring into the conditions of the Irish poor reported that they could not speak favourably of the management of St Patrick's and they referred caustically to its methods of treatment as being 'exclusively moral if that word can be applied to lax discipline, confinement within a certain space and the total absence of all occupation . . .'[37].

But by now the insane were emerging from the neglect and maltreatment of centuries and St Patrick's was entering a new and more enlightened era.

The Beginning of Reform

During the 1790s the prevailing concept of insanity and its treatment was troubling the conscience of various reformers in Western Europe. They rejected the so-called enlightenment which had for so long ordained that insanity was a form of moral weakness requiring methods of treatment based on punishment and terrorisation. Instead they proferred the new and more humane view that irrationality was a product of the pressures of developing civilisation and of the changing social environment; and they argued that the application of disciplinary measures to the insane was a tyranny that deprived them of their natural rights. Foremost, and eventually the most influential, among these reformers were Philippe Pinel of the asylum of Bicêtre in Paris and William Tuke, a Quaker tea-merchant from York. Uninformed of the actions of the other, each was pursuing similar policies of ameliorating the care of the insane. In 1792 Pinel, adopting a new regimen based on kindness, liberated from their chains patients who in some instances had worn them for over thirty years. At the same time Tuke established on similar principles a private asylum in York for members of his own faith[1].

The unshackling of the patients was for the insane an occasion as symbolic as the earlier liberation of the prisoners of the Bastille had been for the wider cause of freedom. They were hardly unrelated events. The French Revolution had created in many hearts a new consciousness of human rights and individual liberty which was to affect political and social institutions generally throughout Western Europe. Gradually other reformers followed the example set by Pinel and Tuke and there was a growing acceptance by those in authority that the problem of providing for the insane should be seen in terms of compassion rather than punishment. This new perception of the care of the insane was also helped by contemporary reforms which were taking place in Western Europe generally in regard to the treatment of criminals. Punishment as a spectacle was ending: the public scaffold gradually disappeared. Many capital offences remained but the carrying out of the death penalty became a private ritual. Conditions in prison, while remaining harsh, improved and prisoners became subject to a more formal regimen than in the past[2]. In this better organised and better supervised system of punishment it became increasingly difficult to justify having the criminal and the lunatic incarcerated together since the latter could hardly be regarded as guilty of a crime. Clearly, if insane persons required to be isolated for their own or the public good then separate places of detention should be provided for them.

The new approach to the insane became known as 'moral treatment' to be carried out in comfortable asylums. Its basic elements were kindness and comfort; irons and chains were rejected except in the most difficult cases and there was an emphasis on treatment, care and exercise. In York the institution was planned to resemble a home with cheerful surroundings. Food was provided liberally:

> . . . a free supply of meat or bread and porter was found of the greatest service at supper in procuring sleep and reducing excitement[3].

For some this treatment had a beneficial outcome which, for a period, led to an unrealistic optimism in regard to the cure of insanity in general. There were, too, other factors in its decline as this account will show.

In Ireland one of the first instances of the impact of the new approach was the foundation in Bloomfield, Dublin, by the Quaker community, of the Retreat for Persons Afflicted with Disorders of the Mind. The decision to build a hospital was taken in 1807; it was opened in 1810 and its programme of care was based on the principles adopted in York. At the end of 1813 the governors were reporting that 'some favourable results have been produced thereby' and while they were 'not discouraged' by the outcome of the treatment given, an air of disappointment runs through their reports. But it could hardly have been otherwise as their records would suggest that many of the patients admitted initially were incurable. While as a general policy all patients were expected to pay for their treatment, and charges varied according to circumstances, in practice some patients were treated free. The governors ensured that there was no discrimination by keeping the manager in ignorance as to those who paid and those who were accepted free. In 1821 the hospital, which is still in existence, decided not to restrict its patients to those of the Quaker faith in the hope of getting more patients in a position to pay a reasonable amount[4].

Hallaran of Cork

The most prominent of the early Irish disciples of moral treatment was William Saunders Hallaran of Cork. He was also the first Irish doctor to write at length on the problems of insanity. In general his writings show that he had deeply studied the origins and therapy of insanity and while many of his beliefs would not be acceptable to-day some of his views are still tenable.

Hallaran was the first physician to the County and City of Cork Lunatic Asylum which developed out of the local house of industry. Like similar institutions elsewhere the latter institution had, originally, no specific accommodation for the insane apart from a few cells. As the demand for the admission of insane persons multiplied the mayor of Cork organised a successful entertainment with the profits of which a new building for twenty-four patients was opened in 1792. Additions to it were made over the subsequent thirty years and by 1822 it had accommodation for three hundred patients. While in effect it was a separate institution from the house of industry it remained under the control of the same governors[5].

Hallaran was physician to the hospital from its opening until 1826. It is not clear when he introduced moral treatment but it is probable that from the beginning he had applied a kindly and humane approach towards the care of his patients for his later writings are those of a compassionate man. His first treatise on the subject of the treatment of the insane, *Practical Observations on the Causes and Cure of Insanity*, did not appear until 1810 and an amended and enlarged version was published eight years later. By 1817 his achievements in the Cork hospital were being publicly acknowledged and Thomas Spring Rice, who was to play a major part in the reform of the care of the insane in Ireland, declared to a parliamentary committee that it was the best managed asylum he had ever seen[6].

Hallaran in his *Observations* suggested that insanity consisted of acute forms which were curable and chronic forms which in general defied the most powerful remedies. Insanity was concerned with 'organic lesions' involving not only the brain but the thoracic and abdominal viscera. There were two basic causes: violent excesses of various kinds and mental pressures such as grief and terror. He cited war, the use of spirituous liquors and 'religious dread' as specific causes.

His treatise dealt with the various forms of therapy in considerable detail. Underlying his whole approach was kindness; if the physician was to be effective in his treatment 'he must be anything but a tyrant'. It was important to talk to the patient and not to argue with him. 'I have invariably made it a rule' he wrote 'to converse with each patient separately . . . on the subject most welcome to his humour'. The results, he claimed, were remarkable.

There were medical and physical therapies which could also be effective in appropriate cases. Bleeding was a remedy to be avoided except in the case of some young persons. The combination of a purgative with an emetic was sometimes beneficial while the utility of antimonial preparations in the acute stage of insanity could not be 'too highly estimated'. Moderate doses of digitalis and opium could also be effective but there was nothing to be gained by blistering. Warm baths were soothing in the convalescent stage of mania and cold shower baths provided relief in certain cases in the early stages of the same condition. Hallaran had a special regard for the circulating swing, a device in use in some of the mental hospitals of the period. It was a type of metal cage in which the patient was suspended after he had been 'sufficiently evacuated with purgative medicines' and swung around for a considerable time[7].

It is clear that while Hallaran was still influenced by some traditional and worthless ideas his emphasis on individual treatment and on discussion with the patient would not be faulted by modern therapists. His successor as physician to the hospital, Thomas Carey Osburne, pursued Hallaran's regimen with enthusiasm, firm in the view that mental disturbance was linked with the disordered state of the abdominal viscera and convinced that this was recognised in the sacred scriptures. He quoted Jeremiah:

> Mine eyes do fail with tears; my bowels are troubled;
> my liver is poured upon the earth.

The liver, according to Osburne, was used metaphorically to express mental perturbation[8].

Osburne, who claimed to have used electric shock treatment successfully, had a number of bizarre patients under his care in the Cork asylum towards the end of the 1820s. They included a sea-captain named Stewart who, when his schooner arrived in Cork from the Barbados in June 1828, was found to have murdered seven of the crew. This he did by beating out the brains of each of them in turn as they entered his cabin; two of the crew who survived had jumped overboard and were picked up by another boat. Stewart was transferred to the Dundrum Criminal Lunatic Asylum after its establishment where, in 1851, he was seen by one of the inspectors of lunacy and described as being then 'a religious monomaniac' still convinced that the crew had meditated mutiny and his death[9]. The doorkeeper of the Cork asylum was for a period a former fisherman who believed that he had been born a salmon and had been caught in a net off Kinsale. He later hanged himself with a strip of blanket after taking the precaution of placing his mattress under him to soften the fall in the event of the strip breaking[10].

Parliamentary moves

The main thrust for reform in Ireland came, not from the medical profession since there were few doctors involved in the care of the insane, but from concerned politicians familiar with existing conditions. Clearly what was required was the ending of the confinement of the insane with criminals and vagrants in the jails and houses of industry and the creation of an asylum system with sufficient accommodation to meet the national demands. There were, fortunately, a sufficient number of individuals interested in the issue who were also active in public life and in a position to set off parliamentary initiatives which culminated in the creation of a network of district lunatic asylums.

In 1804 special provisions for the insane in public institutions amounted only to about 250 places, of which 90 were in the Cork Asylum, 118 in the Dublin House of Industry and most of the remainder in the Waterford and Limerick houses of industry. St Patrick's Hospital was operating mainly as a private institution and there were a few other small privately owned madhouses bringing the number of places in private control to probably less than 200 places. There were in addition hundreds of insane persons incarcerated in jails; but it is probable that the number in confinement in the asylums, jails and other types of accommodation was less than a thousand and that the great bulk of Irish lunatics were wandering at large or confined to peasant cabins or outhouses. A parliamentary committee of 1804 investigating the needs of the aged and infirm poor in Ireland concluded that there was a case for greater provisions for the insane at public expense and recommended that there should be four provincial asylums, one located in Dublin, for 'idiots and lunatics'[11].

However, when in March of the following year Sir John

Newport, who represented Waterford in the House, brought in a bill to give effect to the committee's recommendations there was general opposition to it on the second reading. Members were concerned about the cost of the provisions and unconvinced that there was need for special legislation to provide 'for a thousand mad Irish'. The bill was dropped[12]. Subsequently a minor provision was made in 1806 when an enactment empowered grand juries to raise annually a sum not exceeding one hundred pounds for the support of a lunatic asylum or a ward associated with a house of industry[13]. The paucity of the provision was such that it was generally ignored.

Newport was not easily deterred. He was a staunch Whig noted for the tenacity with which he pursued issues in the Commons and nicknamed 'The Political Ferret' by his parliamentary colleagues[14]. He had, as chairman of the board of governors of Waterford House of Industry, personal knowledge and experience of the shortcomings of existing provisions for the insane and was determined to end them. His perseverance on the subject in parliamentary debates and committees created a momentum towards reform which was later taken up with even greater enthusiasm by a fellow Irish Whig, Thomas Spring Rice, who was not then a member of parliament.

If, however, there appeared to be a general lack of concern about the insane in Ireland the same could largely be said about the position in Britain. The first attention given by the British parliament to the subject was the passage of an Act in 1774 to curb the excesses of private madhouses by providing for their registration and regulation[15]. It remained the only law in regard to the insane until 1808 when new legislation authorised local magistrates in England and Wales to erect public asylums for the poor. It was a permissive, not a compulsory, provision which was greeted with little enthusiasm and by 1827 an asylum had been opened in only nine out of fifty-two counties[16].

That there should have been any legislation at all was due to the reforming zeal of Dr Andrew Halliday who had campaigned, and was to continue to campaign for a considerable period, for a humane provision for the insane both in Britain and Ireland. His views on what was required for Ireland were far more realistic than those of the parliamentary committee of 1804. In a pamphlet published about 1807 he suggested that Ireland required eleven asylums dispersed throughout the country. This suggestion was considered by government commissioners appointed in 1808 to report, *inter alia,* on overcrowding in the Dublin House of Industry. When they reported in the following year they dismissed the practicability of Halliday's suggestion on the grounds that it would be impossible to get enough properly qualified persons to superintend such a relatively large number of asylums and that this would give rise to the risk of mismanagement. The commissioners considered that the best way to meet the problem was by a substantial increase in the accommodation for lunatics in the Dublin House of Industry and by the provision of funds for the expansion of St Patrick's Hospital[17].

Richmond Asylum
The first positive move by the government came in 1810 when, influenced by the report of the previous year, a grant was given to the governors of the Dublin House of Industry to establish a separate asylum 'for the reception of lunatics from all parts of the kingdom'[18]. It was from the government's short-sighted point-of-view a simple and relatively inexpensive solution. Once again Dublin had been made the national centre of care for a group of unwanted and homeless people. Already the Dublin Foundling Hospital was operating in an abominable manner as the repository for many of the country's rejected and abandoned children[19]. Furthermore, the grossly overcrowded house of industry with its national role in regard to the vagrant pauper was failing to cope with the demands for admission from those who flocked into the city from parts of the country where no alternative provision for the poor was available. Now Dublin was also to become the centre for the care of the Irish insane. The hardships and abuses that would inevitably be associated with a single centre

when the great bulk of the population was scattered, rural in character, and far removed from Dublin, was ignored.

Before the new asylum opened in 1815 a special statute established it as an independent institution and provided a separate board of governors. They were appointed by the lord-lieutenant and were obliged to obey all directions given by him[20]. The new institution, now St Brendan's Hospital, Grangegorman, was named after the then lord-lieutenant, the Earl of Richmond and was originally planned to house 218 patients. This was believed to be sufficient to enable the removal of all the lunatics then confined in jails and in the provincial houses of industry and it included forty-two places for those outside the pauper class in a position to make a payment towards their care. It is clear that the authorities in Dublin Castle were somewhat perplexed in trying to settle on the size of the hospital; the chief secretary lacked sufficient information to guide the lord-lieutenant and after the building had begun sought the advice of the governors of the Dublin House of Industry. They had no information apart from the numbers in the various houses of industry. As will be seen the guess then made as to the likely demand was quickly shown to be a gross underestimate[21].

The Richmond Asylum came into existence with certain clear advantages. Alexander Jackson, the physician caring for the insane patients in the house of industry, had taken an interest in it and had in preparation for its opening undertaken a tour of English asylums. His experiences were to have an influence on the design of the hospital and when, appropriately, he was appointed its first medical officer a regimen was implemented based on the principles of moral treatment that he had seen in operation elsewhere. The report prepared by him following his English visit set the atmosphere and the guidelines for the hospital[22]. There was to be an emphasis on the comfort of the patients 'since they are not insensible to the means of comfort or even of enjoyment'. Kind treatment was more effective than 'all the apparatus of chains, darkness (and) anodynes'. It was also important that patients should be classified and accommodated according to their particular degree of insanity in order to facilitate the most effective mode of treatment. Jackson felt strongly that the hospital should be under the control of a resident medical superintendent. In this regard he was in advance of his times. The governors decided that the hospital should be under the general control of a lay manager, referred to as the moral governor; a similar practice was adopted initially in the district lunatic asylums established later.

It was decided as a matter of government policy that the new asylum should be for 'curable' patients only and that the house of industry would look after the 'incurables'. Both would operate on a national basis. All patients seeking admission to either institution were to be screened in the house of industry with a view to deciding where they would be appropriately accommodated. An essential requirement was that each applicant should be accompanied by a certificate of insanity signed by a magistrate, clergyman or doctor[23].

Among the first admissions to the asylum were 120 'curable' patients transferred from the house of industry. But it soon became obvious that any ideas that existed about the probable level of demand had wildly underestimated it. The opening of the new institution had stimulated an overwhelming response; Derry County Infirmary had sent fourteen patients even before its formal opening[24]. From all over Ireland insane persons were being transported to Dublin and were imposing pressures which made it impossible to maintain the type of care which Dr Jackson had set as the ideal. The Richmond Asylum was quickly filled to capacity. In the neighbouring house of industry curable and incurable lunatics continued, as in the past, to share the same accommodation and the same beds as, sane inmates[25]

District lunatic asylums
The fact that the Richmond Asylum was failing to cope with the demands made upon it had come as a surprise and an embarrassment to those who had proposed it in the first instance. Far from meeting a substantial part of the accommodation needs of the country it had merely served to bring

into the open the fact that throughout Ireland there were considerable numbers of insane whose existence was hitherto unknown to the authorities. But if the government had lacked a statistical basis for its planning its advisers had also failed to understand the real nature of insanity. The enthusiasm for moral treatment had given rise to unduly optimistic expectations about what could be achieved in regard to the type of patients previously confined in the jails and houses of industry. It was believed that many such patients would be cured if admitted to asylum treatment in time. It was overlooked, or not understood, that many of these patients were incurable mental defectives who would merely accumulate within the asylum without any expectation of early discharge[26].

There could now be no doubt about the case for further asylums in Ireland. Newport appeared before a parliamentary committee established in 1815 following reported abuses in British asylums and once again argued the case for a better provision for Ireland. He had on this occasion the support of Edward Wakefield, an English Quaker reformer, who had lived in Ireland for two years and who described some of the more harrowing sights involving the insane that he had seen. The committee was clearly influenced by their evidence and when reporting expressed the opinion that the urgency of further provision for the insane Irish was more pressing than English needs[27].

Robert Peel, chief secretary for Ireland, now took the initiative. In 'an animated speech' in the House of Commons in March 1817 he deplored the lack of provision in Ireland and secured agreement to the establishment of yet another committee to look specifically at the Irish situation[28]. Once again witnesses came forward to describe in graphic detail the horrors associated with the care of lunatics in Ireland. The most compelling evidence on this occasion was given by Thomas Spring Rice (to whom reference has already been made) a Limerick landlord, who could speak with authority as a governor of the local house of industry where lunatics were housed in particularly vile conditions. The committee was as convinced as its predecessor about the need for action but was more specific about what should be done. It recommended that, in addition to the Richmond and Cork asylums, there should be four or five asylums each serving specified districts and capable of accommodating 120 to 150 patients. The basis of care in the institutions should be moral treatment, the committee being satisfied that it was more successful than what it referred to as 'casual medical prescription'. It also suggested that unwanted public buildings such as army barracks could be used as asylums[29].

On this occasion there was quick action. William Vesey Fitzgerald, a former chancellor of the Irish exchequer, introduced a bill drafted by Spring Rice that quickly became law[30]. It gave power to the lord-lieutenant to direct the erection of whatever number of asylums he thought appropriate along the lines recommended by the committee. The grand juries were empowered to raise funds for them but there would also be support from central government sources. While the asylums would be under the local direction of governors appointed by the lord-lieutenant their planning and establishment would be the responsibility of a special central authority known as the Commissioners for General Control and Correspondence. This initial legislation was amended in minor respects by an Act of 1820[31]. Both Acts were repealed in 1821 when they were consolidated and further amended by new legislation again drafted by Spring Rice who by now had become a Whig member of parliament for County Limerick. Its main provisions were similar to those of the original Act and with some later minor amendments it became the basis on which the Irish lunatic asylum system was established and developed[32].

The commissioners given the task of establishing the asylums had been appointed in 1817[33]. They consisted of eight members, four medical and four lay. Subject to the approval of the lord-lieutenant their task was to decide on the location and dimensions of the new institutions and on the districts to be served by them. Their responsibilities also included the making of arrangements for design and construction but their involvement ceased once an asylum opened its doors to patients. Decisions about the most suitable location were not easy and the commissioners were subject to many representations from local interests. When, for instance, they decided that in the first instance one asylum would be adequate for the province of Ulster, located either in Belfast or Armagh, they were subjected to pressures advocating the special claims of the Belfast area. A petition from the Belfast Incorporated Charitable Society drew attention to the large number of lunatic poor in that city and in the event the commissioners recommended the establishment of an asylum in both Armagh and Belfast[34].

By 1830 the district lunatic asylum system was taking shape; four new asylums had been completed at costs varying between £21,000 and £30,000. They were Armagh, Limerick, Belfast and Derry. In addition sites had been chosen for asylums at Maryborough and Carlow and a proposal to establish one at Ballinasloe was awaiting a decision of the lord-lieutenant. Each of the new asylums was to serve a wide region; for example, that at Armagh was intended to serve Counties Monaghan, Cavan, Fermanagh, and Armagh and the Ballinasloe centre was intended for the whole of Connaught[35].

The political and social background

The awakening of government concern for the insane in the early nineteenth century was not an isolated development. Fundamental changes were taking place in the whole social order which were influencing not only the way men lived but their relationships with each other. The industrial revolution, the movement to the towns, the rapidly increasing populations, were giving rise to new social issues and problems. In the matter of government there were threats to the old order. Ominous political philosophies concerned with the rights of man were sowing ideas of equality and freedom in the hearts of the lower orders. There was a further challenge to traditional privileges in the emerging middle classes, people whose wealth and prominence derived not from their birth but from the opportunities for advancement in the new economic environment. In various parts of Europe attacks on the political power for so long distributed between monarchy and aristocracy were leading to a growing acceptance by the ruling classes that self-preservation, if nothing more altruistic, required some concessions to the poor and the powerless.

Where Ireland was concerned there were also indigenous influences at work. A combination of political and social factors had created a bleak and threatening national landscape. The insurrection of 1798, the repressive measures that followed it, the illusory prospects promised by Castlereagh, Pitt and the other protagonists of the Union had all incited public unrest. Violence was growing. A rapidly increasing population was leading to deteriorating social conditions. Work was scarce and becoming scarcer.

The landlords in general were not interested in improving their estates and gave little employment; industry failed to develop to any significant degree. Destitution had become the common lot. Between 1800 and 1830 various parliamentary committees had considered the needs of the Irish poor but all baulked at the prospect of providing a system of poor laws suitable for Irish circumstances. Since the rights of property were regarded as paramount any broad social provision requiring additional taxation would have posed an unacceptable threat. Help for the poor in general would merely encourage pauperism among what was regarded as a work-shy population. A parliamentary committee of 1830 warned that, 'a false step may here be of such fatal consequences that it greatly behoves the legislature to proceed cautiously'[36].

Yet, so long as violence was not done to the just rights of property, there was a desire to make some gestures of benevolence to the largely dissident population. The alternative would have been continued dependence on repression which would almost certainly lead eventually to calamity. Consequently, there was gradual if reluctant progress towards the grant of full emancipation to Catholics. Government support for the charter schools and foundling hospitals, elements in the machinery devised by the nineteenth century Protestant ascendancy for extirpating Irish Catholicism, was reduced and eventually dropped to the general approbation of the majority population[37].

While a line was drawn at making any broad effort to alleviate the widespread poverty there was, nevertheless, by the early years of the century, a considerable, if uneven, provision of services for the sick poor. On the face of it, at least, Ireland was more advanced than Britain in government-supported welfare provisions. Dublin had a considerable provision of hospitals dating mainly from the eighteenth century when they were founded and supported largely by benevolent members of the merchant and professional classes. They included Dr Steevens Hospital; the Charitable Infirmary (Jervis Street); Mercer's Hospital; the Meath Hospital; the Rotunda Lying-In Hospital; the Hospital for Incurables and St Patrick's Hospital. Added to these during the first three decades of the nineteenth century were Cork Street Fever Hospital; Sir Patrick Dun's Hospital; the Westmoreland Lock Hospital; the National Eye Hospital (later Royal Victoria Eye and Ear Hospital); the Institution for Sick Children (later National Children's Hospital) and the Coombe Lying-In Hospital. Further voluntary hospitals were established in the 1830s notably the Adelaide Hospital, the Royal City of Dublin Hospital and the first religious controlled general hospital, St Vincent's Hospital. In addition the Dublin House of Industry, while still basically an institution for vagrants, contained a number of hospital units called after the viceroys who held office at the time of their construction, Hardwicke, Richmond and Whitworth[38].

Outside Dublin a number of voluntary hospitals had also come into existence, notably the North and South Infirmaries in Cork; and St John's Hospital and Barrington's Hospital in Limerick[39]. But in general, the provincial areas lacked the benevolent middle classes who were the strength and inspiration of the early voluntary hospital system. The rural poor had to be content with the limited provision of the county infirmaries established in 1765 by the old Irish parliament when the expanding Dublin hospital system had served to draw attention to the lack of services for the remainder of the country[40]. Funded by grand jury presentments and private contributions they were, under the pre-Union government, little more than a gesture. John Howard, the British prison and hospital reformer, who visited many of them about 1787 found that they were then mostly wretched places, short of funds, dirty, over-crowded and in a state of disrepair[41]. However, under the reformed administrative and social provisions of the post-Union years a gradual improvement took place in them. Reports prepared for the commissioners investigating Irish poverty in the early 1830s referred favourably to most of the twenty-three infirmaries then in existence although the investigators were critical of the extent to which they had become centres for chronic rather than acutely ill patients[42].

There was also a widespread provision of fever hospitals, an essential social requirement in a period of frequent epidemics that lacked any scientific understanding of coping with contagion other than by isolation. By 1830 there were seventy-four separate fever hospitals supported by private subscriptions and county presentments. Some were minimal in character; the twelve-bedded hospital in Mallow consisted of a timber shed thrown against a wall at a cost of £20[43]. But the treatment of the sick, including those with fever, in rural Ireland depended to a large extent at this period on the local dispensary doctor, if there happened to be one. Because the county infirmary service was so limited, Acts of 1805 and 1818 had empowered grand juries to contribute to public dispensaries[44]. Reports during 1817 and 1818 on a fever outbreak consisting of a combination of dysentery and typhus show that in many areas cases among the poor were treated by dispensary doctors. Some of the doctors themselves fell victims to the fever[45]. Evidence given during the poverty investigations of the early 1830s show that by then many, but not all, parts of the country had a dispensary doctor. Some of them appear to have had no formal qualifications; but at least three-quarters of the doctors had been trained in Britain. British-trained doctors were debarred from posts in the county infirmaries which were reserved for physicians and surgeons who had graduated from the Dublin medical schools. This statutory regulation was resented by many of the dispensary doctors and they actively competed against the infirmaries not only for patients but for subscriptions[46].

In addition to the provision of institutions and dispensaries Ireland had, at this period, the advantage of notable medical schools, a good supply of doctors, and a distinguished and self-confident medical *élite* some of whom were winning international recognition. The high teaching standards and research achievements of the Royal College of Physicians, the Royal College of Surgeons, the medical school of Trinity College, and the Dublin hospitals associated with them were widely acknowledged. Irish surgeons and physicians of the period such as Abraham Colles, John Cheyne, Robert Graves and William Stokes were perpetuating their names by their contributions to medical science[47].

While the advancement and distribution of medical care was still seen as a matter largely for voluntary initiatives and private subscriptions the government had clearly accepted that it, too, had a role and a responsibility. Its involvement was, of course, subject to the overall policy of *laissez-faire* and the eternal vigilance of the taxable classes. As yet they had no cause for alarm; the extent of the demands of sickness on the public purse was quite modest. An Act of 1806 provided for the regulation of county infirmaries and other public hospitals by requiring them to make annual returns of their accounts and details of the numbers of patients treated[48]. A firm policy was established in regard to those seeking public funding. It was seen as primarily a matter for local taxation and grants did not normally exceed the equivalent of receipts from private subscriptions. Where it was improbable that a charity could be maintained in that manner, direct parliamentary grants could be given but they were strictly limited to Dublin charities.[49]. This was a recognition that Dublin institutions bore a considerable part of the burden of Irish poverty in the absence of adequate provisions in many rural areas. But even then there were limitations on what the government was prepared to pay; during the early 1830s wards were closed in some of the Dublin hospitals for lack of funds[50].

The principle of government intervention on behalf of the sick was, therefore, well established in the early years of the nineteenth century; enabling legislation had been enacted and a considerable number of institutions and dispensaries were in existence even if, qualitively and quantitively, they may have had short comings. MacDonagh has written:

> If one takes policy and structure as the criteria Ireland had one of the most advanced health services in Europe in the first half of the nineteenth century[51].

Obviously the creation of humane facilities for the insane could also be contemplated particularly since, as the government wrongly believed, the numbers were very small and the financial implications likely to be of no great consequence. Special measures for pauper lunatics were unlikely to increase lunacy. In such a favourable atmosphere it was not surprising that the main protagonists of lunacy reform in Ireland were successful in bringing about more rapid change than in Britain. They were, in any event, assiduous and well placed individuals. Robert Peel, chief secretary for Ireland from 1812 to 1818, recognised the need for change and was in a position to facilitate it. While in office he was, in effect, a one-man cabinet with the authority and the determination to implement quickly measures which, in his view, would help to reduce the level of social unrest in Ireland. He had, in particular, advanced the freeing of public administration from the dominance of political bias. A new type of government administration was taking form. Senior public officials were emerging who for the first time were bringing a considerable degree of impartiality to their judgments on contending parties and social issues[52].

As has been shown, Peel was responsible for the establishment of the select committee of 1817 that led to the initial legislation for the establishment of district asylums. Furthermore, Newport's persistence ensured that the government would not forget about the Irish insane and he gave the campaign for reform its early momentum. But it is to Spring

Rice that most of the credit must go. His contemporary, the notable reformer Sir Andrew Halliday, asserted that the introduction of district asylums into Ireland was due 'to the indefatigable exertions and persevering zeal of Mr. Thomas Spring Rice, the worthy member for Limerick'[53]. As already noted Spring Rice was active in drawing attention to the short-comings in the provision for the Irish insane before he became a parliamentarian. When eventually he entered parliment in 1820 he quickly and successfully brought about the strengthening and extension of the original legislation enabling the establishment of district asylums. During his subsequent career as a Whig politician he took advantage of the fact that he was strategically placed politically to ensure the continued development and improvement of the system. In 1827 he was under-secretary for the Home Department (which directed the Irish administration) in Canning's government and soon after taking up duty he was prodding the officials in Dublin Castle to ensure that action was being taken under the lunacy legislation[54]. After a period in opposition he took office again as secretary to the treasury from 1830 to 1834 in Lord Grey's administration and became chancellor of the exchequer the following year under Lord Melbourne. He held that post until 1839 when he retired almost entirely from public life on being created Baron Monteagle[55].

While Spring Rice was clearly concerned for the insane he was firmly opposed like many of his political contemporaries to a poor law for Ireland. Writing to Dr John Doyle, Bishop of Kildare and Leighlin in 1829 he expressed the view that 'relief without work is mischievous in every point of view. A promise or even an endeavour by the State to provide work is vain, fruitless and can only end in disappointment'. But he believed that support for the sick, the insane and the disabled was justified[56].

In arguing the case for Irish lunatic asylums he had persistently pointed to conditions in Limerick House of Industry as exemplifying the gross defects in the existing arrangements. When eventually it was decided that Limerick should have one of the first of the new asylums he personally supervised the planning of it. He had initial drawings made which he discussed with doctors and architects and later developed into more detailed proposals that he placed before the Commissioners for Superintendence and Correspondence responsible for the planning of the system. After the asylum had been built he proudly claimed that he had never seen a better building for the money[57]. In view of his efforts on behalf of the insane of Ireland he had, one feels, earned the right to his piece of self-congratulation. Nevertheless, the design of his asylum was not particularly imaginative; like others of the early period, it still retained jail-like characteristics. As will be seen, the concept of later district asylums moved more firmly towards being hospitals in appearance and lay-out.

The Asylum System Expands

The trend that had become apparent after the opening of the first district asylum continued and the number of insane seeking admission increased steadily. At the beginning of 1837 there were over 1,600 lunatics in the overcrowded district institutions and another 1,500 in the jails, houses of industry and private asylums[1]. By 1843 there were 2,028 patients occupying accommodation intended for 1,220 in the asylums. Others were being looked after in a variety of small local institutions which, the parliamentary committee of that year reported, were 'miserable and inadequate' and provided 'a coercive and severe system of treatment'. There were still degrading and bizarre sights. White, the inspector, visiting the small asylum associated with Wexford House of Industry saw a naked patient surrounded by straw chained to a wall; two others, trying to warm themselves, were stretched on top of a metal grill protecting a fireplace. They were, he reported, the most frightful cases he had ever seen. Both the male and female keeper were incapable of discharging their duties[2].

Faced with a considerable amount of similar evidence of this sort the committee had little choice but to recommend a substantial expansion of the existing district asylum system. This could be done in a number of ways; by increasing the number of asylums, by expanding existing premises or by providing separate institutions for those referred to as idiots and incurables. This expansion would not only reduce the overcrowding in the existing asylums but serve to end admissions of lunatics to the gaols and union workhouses, neither of which the committee regarded as a fit setting for their care[3]. Furthermore a large number of other mentally disturbed persons, calculated by the Royal Irish Constabulary in 1844 to total 6,217, were still roaming the country, unwanted and unprotected[4]. An English visitor to Mayo about this time described how a wandering mad woman rushed into a cabin he was visiting, snatched a glass of grog, and ran away 'laughing and jabbering Irish . . . the filthiest, most ragged, most squalid of her sex, her dark hair streaming down her smoke-browned neck, her black eyes bright with partial madness . . .'[5].

The government now launched an expansion of the asylum system of ever-growing dimensions which was to continue until the end of the century. At an early stage some consideration was given to the concept of a large separate asylum for incurable patients in each of the provinces with the district asylums reserved for those regarded as curable[6]. This notion came to nothing probably because the 130 union workhouses opened between 1840 and 1845 offered too tempting an opportunity to provide for many of the incurable without additional cost to the tax payers. Thus, despite occasional protestations about the unsuitability of workhouses for the care of the insane, curable or incurable, policy during the next fifty years was based on expanding the district lunatic asylum system while at the same time using the workhouses to provide some relief.

Between 1845 and 1853 Carlow, Maryborough, Limerick, Clonmel, Waterford, Belfast, Armagh, Derry, and the Richmond Asylums were all extended and new asylums were opened in Mullingar (1855), Cork (1852, to replace the existing asylum), Killarney (1852), Sligo (1855), Omagh (1853) and Kilkenny (1852)[7]. A further series of new asylums was opened in the 1860s: Downpatrick (1865), Castlebar (1866), Letterkenny (1866), Ennis (1868), Enniscorthy (1868) and Monaghan (1869). A proposal to build a new asylum at Nenagh was dropped when it was decided on grounds of

economy to expand the existing asylum at Clonmel by acquir-
ing a neighbouring workhouse building. The new building was
operated as a separate asylum for about eight years until its
administration was integrated with that of the parent asylum
in 1860[8].

Apart from Antrim (1899) no further new institutions
were established before the end of the century but there was
a continuous process expanding the existing buildings. By
1901 there were almost 17,000 inmates in asylums originally
planned for less than 5,000 and the total insane population
then in institutions or at large was calculated at over 25,000.
The estimation of lunatics 'at large' was made annually by
members of the Royal Irish Constabulary. Although in no
way competent to do so, every policeman was required to
adjudge the number of insane in his district. His assessments
were usually based on hearsay knowledge or popular opinions
that a person was 'harmless' or 'a softy'. In view of the lack
of definition of insanity it is unlikely that a more professional
view would have arrived at a significantly different total. In
any event it was clear that the burden of insanity in Ireland
had become a remarkably heavy one. Fifty years earlier the
number of known insane was less than 10,000. Now with a
smaller population the number was two-and-a-half times
more; about 56 for every 100,000 of the population compared with 41 in England and Wales and 45 in Scotland[9].

The asylum buildings

The earlier asylums built before the dissolution in 1835 of
the original central board consisted of a radiating building of
two storeys with exercise yards confined to irregular spaces
between the radii, the front building and an outer wall.
Examples of these buildings are still to be seen in Waterford
and Ballinasloe. They were cluttered and dreary in character,
lacking in ventilation and abyssmally short of such basic
facilities as baths, closets and kitchen accommodation. It
was clear that the ideas of the central board about the type
of setting necessary for the care of lunatics were anchored in
the past. These early buildings were more in keeping with

the creation of a jail-like, secure complex of buildings, where the emphasis was on confinement and isolation[10].

In 1835 the Board of Works took over the responsibility of the former central board for the provision of asylum buildings. By then not only were the shortcomings of the earlier asylums recognised but the Board had a better understanding of the therapeutic and caring intentions of the asylums.

Frederick Villiers Clarendon, one of the Board's architects, described in 1849 the basis on which future asylums were being planned:

> I have proceeded on the principle that lunatic asylums are hospitals for recovery of curable patients and houses for the reception of incurable lunatics and not prisons for the safe-custody of dangerous mad-men and with this view I would propose to abolish as far as it is practicable any arrangement that may present the gaol-like character of many of the existing asylums...[11]

Clarendon's vision of the new concept asylum was arrived at without any consultation with the inspectors of lunacy. In theory there was supposed to be close working co-operation between them; in practice there was little communication or harmony[12]. Nugent, one of the inspectors, told a parliamentary committee in 1855 that the Board of Works never consulted the inspectors about the general design of the buildings although there was some discussion about the internal arrangements[13]. It is doubtful whether a closer liaison would have made any difference. There is no evidence that Nugent, or his colleague White, had any particular ideas about asylum design. Neither had the professional knowledge or experience of value on which to base an informed view. In these early days of the asylum system there were few precedents and little expert knowledge so that one man's guess was as good as another's. The overriding aim, shared by all involved, was to create a setting in which patients could be cared for in a more humane manner than hitherto. Some ideas were, however, borrowed from asylums in Britain which had been viewed by John Radcliffe, a member of the

Board of Works, accompanied by an architect[14].

The asylums established in the 1850s and 1860s were therefore somewhat different in character from their predecessors. Examples are to be seen in Cork (the present asylum replaced Hallaran's original asylum), Mullingar, Sligo, Omagh and Monaghan. They were mainly three storey buildings, gothic in style, with a fair amount of architectural ornamentation and innovation including, for effect, projecting day-rooms. They were usually sited on the outskirts of larger towns, sometimes strikingly located on raised ground such as in Cork and Enniscorthy so that they dominated the surrounding area. Most of them had prime land attached which was used not only to provide work for the inmates, many of farming origin, but also food for the institution. The prison-like elements of the earlier buildings were dropped although there was still a considerable degree of security associated with them. The Board of Works decided that the enclosing walls should be no more than six and a half feet high; the exercise yards were planned in a more open manner and the iron bars disappeared from the windows.

It was inevitable that there would be some reaction from the tax-payers still smarting under the costs of the poor law system. The necessary finance for the buildings came in the first instance from the central consolidated fund but had to be repaid half-yearly through a compulsory presentment in each county for which the grand jury was responsible[15]. There were suggestions of extravagance in relation to the decorative features of the buildings and allegations of defects in the accommodation which led to an investigation by a group of treasury commissioners at the end of 1855. In general they were satisfied with what had been done. They reported that the buildings were pleasing in style and built, 'in a manner highly creditable to the architects engaged and ornamental to the country'. While they acknowledged that there might have been too much embellishment at Cork and Sligo and, to a lesser extent, in Killarney and Mullingar, they found an anxiety on the part of asylum governors to avoid the bare, forbidding character of the poor-law workhouses so that the new asylums 'should not reflect too much the poverty, crime and misfortunes of the country'[16].

If aesthetically the outward appearance of the asylums was reasonably pleasing there were, on the other hand, internal defects. In all the buildings there was considerable damp rising from the failure to fill properly the wall joints with mortar. Heating was inadequate. In some instances dormitories were far bigger than intended because the directions of the Board of Works about having sufficient single rooms for one-third of the patients were ignored. Large dormitories were in general keeping with the depersonalised environment of the Victorian pauper institution whether it was an orphanage, workhouse, hospital or asylum. The expense of providing otherwise would have been formidable. Nevertheless, where the asylums were concerned, it would have been reasonable to expect greater emphasis on small dormitories given the notions of close personal attention implicit in the concept of moral treatment. However, the large bare dormitory lacking any furniture but closely packed beds, often accommodating fifty or more patients, became not only a feature of the nineteenth century asylum but a legacy for the twentieth century that some of the existing mental hospitals still have not succeeded in rejecting.

Development of private asylums

The development of the district asylums stimulated the contemporaneous growth of private asylums. The restriction of the district institutions to pauper patients served to emphasise the shortage of accommodation for those in a position to pay. At the beginning of the century only a few small private asylums existed. Dr Hallaran had opened Citadella, near Cork in 1799; Dr Boate owned a small establishment at Portobello, Dublin; and there were also asylums in Downpatrick and Carlow. All were operated as businesses by individual proprietors. There were almost certainly others. While the Prisons Act of 1787 had given the inspector-general of prisons the authority to visit all places where the insane were detained the activities of these profit-making enterprises were largely ignored. As already mentioned, St Patrick's Hospital, contrary to its charter, was also admitting private patients and with Bloomfield Retreat provided about 100 private places in the 1820s[17].

Between 1800 and 1830 the gross abuses of private madhouses in Britain were the subject of various committees and private member bills in a largely apathetic British parliament. When in 1814 a private member bill proposed regulating English madhouses a committee of the Royal College of Physicians in Ireland that included James Cleghorne, physician to St Patrick's Hospital, urged that its provisions be extended to Ireland. The Bill would have established commissioners to oversee the institutions with, *inter alia*, the power to direct the discharge of patients. The Irish committee had some reservations about this particular provision 'on account of the art and cunning so frequently practised by insane persons by which some of the most experienced practitioners have at times been deceived'[18]. However the proposers of the Bill opposed extending it to Ireland because it was framed for England where the madhouses were 'so superior' and because the controls proposed would be too expensive and quite unsuitable for Ireland[19]. Since the accounts of the English private madhouses of the period make grim reading it is hard to visualise the conditions of those in Ireland. In any event the Bill failed to get through parliament.

In 1823 in addition to St Patrick's Hospital and Bloomfield Retreat there were at least three small private asylums in Dublin all located in the Finglas area[20]. Finglas was to remain the main location for this type of institution. It had earlier been a fashionable residential district but had felt the impact of the social and political changes that followed the Union when many ascendancy families moved abroad. By the 1840s Finglas village was being described as 'amongst the poorest and most destitute in the empire' and some of its former mansions had been converted into asylums[21].

When the legislation aimed at reforming the Irish prison system was enacted in 1826 it contained a number of provisions directed at private asylums. They required the inspector-general of prisons to visit and report once every two years on every madhouse kept for profit. Penalties were prescribed for persons molesting or obstructing a visiting inspector. No other statutory controls were imposed until legislation of 1842 provided for the grant of licences on an annual basis at quarter sessions by justices of the peace subject to revocation by the lord chancellor. Patients could be detained only on the basis of a certificate signed by two doctors; certain records had to be kept and where the asylum was not actually under the direction of a doctor there had to be a visiting physician. The private asylums now became subject to six-monthly visits by the inspectors of lunacy[22] .

The establishment of a compulsory registration system revealed the position about the number of private asylums actually operating. By 1844 there were fourteen licensed premises. Seven of these were in the Dublin area and the others were in Cork, Limerick, Armagh and Queen's County (Laoighis)[23]. Private asylums like the public asylums were under constant pressure for admissions. By the end of 1862 there were twenty-one private asylums caring for over five hundred patients[24]. Among the first centres to be registered was Hampstead House in Glasnevin which had been in operation since 1821. Later an adjoining sister institution, Highfield House, was developed. Both these institutions still remain in existence under the direction of the medical family, the Eustaces, who founded them and who had also been associated with the establishment of Bloomfield Retreat[25]. Later in the century St Vincent's Hospital, Fairview, Dublin (1857), the Stewart Institution (1869), St John of God Hospital (1882) and St Patrick's, Belmont Park, Waterford (1882) were the most notable additions. By the early years of the twentieth century the total number of places in the private institutions had increased to about 800 through extensions to the existing buildings rather than the opening of new institutions[26].

It is not possible to generalise about the quality of care given in the nineteenth century private asylums since they varied considerably in size, organisation and motivation. Conditions in St Patrick's were frequently the subject of criticism largely because of the limitation of its site and the fact that its plan was based on mid-eighteenth century notions of caring for the insane. The religious-controlled institutions such as Bloomfield Retreat and St Vincent's (Daughters of Charity), which were charitable in motivation, were well conducted and not subject to serious defects. This cannot be said of all the smaller houses operated on a profit-making basis mainly by individual doctors. While it is clear that those intended for the particularly well-to-do, such as Hampstead House, always maintained a high level of care most of the other private asylums were merely centres of detention with spartan standards of accommodation for those who could not afford better.

The inspectors were, nevertheless, remarkably tolerant and sparing in their criticism. In 1851 they were 'happy' about the general state of the private asylums and of the view that the majority of complaints made against them were 'fanciful in their origin' and arose principally from 'delusions connected with family feuds'. Two years later they commented on the 'humane and judicious manner' in which the asylums were, for the most part, conducted. Nugent, reporting alone in 1857, admitted that some of them were inferior but noted signs of improvement. He explained that the defects arose from the fact that the proprietors lacked capital and that the patients paid irregularly. But he reported that there was no evidence of cruelty in them and defended the institutions because, he claimed, without them, their patients would have been neglected. He expressed similar views in the following year in evidence to the government commission of enquiry examining the state of Irish asylums in general[27].

The commissioners were far more critical. They found that some of the asylums were not fit to be licensed. They reported that sometimes the amount paid by the patient or his friends was 'miserably small' and that to ensure adequate profits patients were subjected to considerable restraints so that fewer staff would be required. St Patrick's Hospital, too, was found wanting. The visiting committee there had given up visiting. The lone bath for one hundred and fifty patients had been out of order for several months at the time of the visit of the commissioners; and there was inadequate heating and poor ventilation[28].

The inspectors were undoubtedly at a disadvantage in supervising the private asylums in that they did not represent the licensing authority. The commission of 1858 recognised this and recommeded that the licensing responsibility be transferred from the various quarter sessions to the central lunacy board. But this was not done; the only influence that the inspectors continued to have on the grant or regrant of licences was to submit copies of their visiting reports to the magistrates[29].

There is no evidence that, given greater authority, the inspectors would have adopted a tougher approach. Their reports continued to be mildly critical. In 1868 they regarded some of the institutions as 'poorly arranged and imperfectly carried on yet without any glaring defect to call for condemnation or censure'[30]. Low standards which would not have been tolerated elsewhere were obviously acceptable to the inspectors. George Tucker, an Australian doctor and proprietor of a private asylum, wrote after a visit to Hartfield House, Drumcondra, 'the place had a neglected air and was altogether repulsive'[31]. Questioned by a parliamentary committee in 1877, Nugent strongly defended the Irish private asylums. He never recollected the suspension of any of them during his thirty years as inspector. He had only once, he said, to complain to the lord chancellor and this was about personal abuse he received from one proprietor. Furthermore he considered that 'no underhand work' was being perpetrated in any of the asylums and he had never heard of a case of wrongful or wilful detention in any of them[32].

Nugent had been less than candid if not actually untruthful. He was the dominant of the two inspectors of lunacy and had shown throughout his official career a noted reluctance to become involved in criticism of medical colleagues particularly if they were influential members of the profession. Burdett, writing in 1891, after Nugent and his long-term colleague, Hatchell, had ceased to be inspectors, referred to their 'meagre and rosy-tinted generalities' in reports on the private asylums[33]. Sometimes unpleasant facts were concealed by them of which a notable example was that involving Dr William Harty.

Harty was a prominent member of the medical profession who held in addition to other appointments that of physician to the Dublin prisons. He was also proprietor of a private asylum, Finglas House. Following the enactment of the legislation of 1842 which subjected the asylums to registration Harty emerged as spokesman for the proprietors and addressed a pamphlet to the chief secretary, Robert Peel. It protested indignantly against official interference in private institutions on the basis that they were in general well conducted and under the control of doctors[34]. But even then there were doubts about the way Harty himself was operating his asylum. In 1842 following court proceedings the lord chancellor had directed him to release a woman patient after his refusal to allow visits to her by a doctor and by her brother Sir Nicholas Chinnery[35]. About ten years later further court proceedings revealed that Harty had seduced another woman patient and that their son had grown up in the asylum[36]. This must have been particularly embarrassing for the inspectors whose duties required them to inspect the asylum every six months. In 1854 Finglas House disappeared quietly from the list of private asylums in their annual report without any comment by them or any report of the case.

The views of the man who held the post of chief clerk of the lunacy office, and who would have been a close colleague of the inspectors during part of their stewardship, are of interest. W.J. Corbett was chief clerk during the 1850s and 1860s and later served as a Parnellite member of parliament for twelve years. He became personally interested in the advancement of the care of the insane and in 1893 gave his views on the subject of private asylums to an international congress in Chicago[37]. His opposition to them was clear. While he conceded that some of them were 'good, kind, philanthropic, conscientious and deserving of confidence' his experience had turned him against private asylums in general. He said:

> It is the original sin of the system under which, for pecuniary consideration, not only the unsound but frequently the sane are shut up, and kept in the custody of speculators who carry on a trade in lunatics, that excites my aversion and deadly hostility.

He claimed that for a consideration it was easy to obtain a medical certificate establishing the insanity of a relative and that this was being done for a variety of motives including revenge; punishment for misconduct, reckless extravagance, dissipation and acts of immorality; or simply for 'disgracing the family name'.

Corbett described a case which appeared to have happened in the early 1880s. A jealous wife succeeded in having a philandering husband detained without communication in a private asylum for two years. A writ of *habeas corpus* eventually secured his discharge. Corbett quoted the *Irish Times* as having commented at the time:

> we feel called to express our opinion that private lunatic asylums should not be tolerated in a free state.

In general it must be said that there is no evidence of gross or widespread abuse either of the law or in the care of patients in the Irish private asylums of the period. There was clearly a public demand for them arising largely from the fact that the district lunatic asylums were operated as pauper institutions. When, later, provision was made for the admission to the latter of private patients it did not, however, change the inferior social standing which the district lunatic asylums had by then acquired in the minds of the class-conscious middle and upper classes. While the very well-to-do among them could afford to pay for a good private asylum, the less wealthy sought a more basic institution. The standards in some of these cheaper institutions were very low indeed, and were encouraged by the ease with which licences could be obtained and by the over-tolerant attitude of the inspectors.

There were, however, fewer complaints about them from the 1890s onwards although no significant changes were made in the statutory controls over the private asylums until 1945[38].

Administering and Staffing the Asylums

It was fortunate for the care of the insane that the development of the district asylums was well under way before the Irish poor law system was initiated by the Poor Relief Act of 1838. The workhouses for which it provided were harsh and forbidding in character, planned deliberately to facilitate the creation of an 'irksome' and unsympathetic environment where paupers would have no inclination to dally at the expense of the ratepayer. If the workhouses had emerged before the asylums it would be difficult to envisage the government doing other than choosing on grounds of economy and administrative convenience to provide for the care of the insane as part of a unified system under the direction of the local boards of poor law guardians. In such a setting the emphasis would almost certainly have been on the pauperism of the inmates rather than their insanity, the financial resources would have been much more limited, and the quality of care of a lower standard.

The commission established in 1830 under Archbishop Whately to report on the needs of the Irish poor had, in fact, recommended that the asylums be brought under the direction of the Poor Law Commissioners[1]. The views of the Whately commission in general were rejected by the government in favour of those of George Nicholls, the English poor law commissioner, who had been called on in 1836 to devise a poor law system more in keeping with the dominant *laissez-faire* views of the period. Nicholls advised the government to continue in existence a separate administration for the asylums but suggested nevertheless that 'pauper idiots and lunatics not in a dangerous state' be cared for in the work-houses[2].

Six years later when the building of one hundred and thirty workhouses was well under way, Nicholls, who was directing their construction in great detail, informed the chief secretary that they would contain a total of 2,300 places for idiots and lunatics. He was now clearly unhappy about accommodating them in the workhouses and suggested that it would be better if their needs were met by adding chronic wards to the district asylums[3]. But such a change in policy would have required time and there was now no way in which he could prevent the workhouses becoming the repositories for large numbers of insane people. By 1845 there were only ten district asylums in existence with about 1,300 places. On the other hand all parts of the country had available a local workhouse which, despite its spartan and oppressive atmosphere, quickly became in the prevailing famine conditions a haven for the whole range of human misery. The introduction of the asylums had brought out demands far in excess of what had been anticipated; now the workhouses were giving a further stimulus to the un-covering of a more realistic picture of Irish insanity. The asylum came generally to be regarded as the appropriate centre for those believed to be the curable insane and for those designated, often unjustifiably, dangerous patients; the workhouse dealt with the remainder, in most instances the congenitally mentally defective or, as they were called, the idiots and the imbeciles. The central lunacy adminis-tration became responsible for overseeing the well-being of those in both institutions although it had little influence or power in relation to workhouse conditions.

Central lunacy administration

It could not be said that there was a strong central adminis-tration to guide the development of services for the insane until after the departure of the British administration from

Ireland and the assignment of responsibility in this area to the new Department of Local Government[4]. Until then the asylums remained under the general control of the lord-lieutenant acting through the inspectors of lunacy and a board of control which, throughout the period, varied in constitution and authority.

The unpaid eight-man board established in 1817 had been given no functions other than arranging for the building of the first few district lunatic asylums. It went out of existence in 1835 when it was supposed that all the asylums likely to be required had been provided. The Commissioners of the Board of Works then took over as a board of control also limited in function to maintaining and providing buildings and without any say or responsibility in the management of the institutions or the care of patients[5]. In 1860 in an effort to co-ordinate the functions of the Board of Works and those of the inspectors of lunacy a new body with broader functions than its predecessor, known as the Commissioners of General Control and Correspondence, was established[6]. Its members included the chairman of the Board of Works and the two inspectors of lunacy. But it served little purpose; the Board of Works continued independently to decide matters relating to buildings while the inspectors gave their advice to the government on other lunacy matters[7].

In 1891 a committee established by the lord-lieutenant to review the then central administration rejected suggestions that the Local Government Board might become responsible for lunacy matters. It considered that the Board already had too wide a variety of responsibilities and, in any event, believed that the asylum system needed a separate administration. It proposed, as an interim improvement, a board of control similar to that originally provided for seventy years previously. The board would include the chairman of the Board of Works, the two inspectors of lunacy and other undesignated persons. The functions assigned to it would relate to the district asylums only and not to insane in other institutions. For the longer term, however, the committee, largely influenced by the position in Scotland, recommended legislation to create a General Board of Commissioners of Lunacy in Ireland. It would have five to seven members, including the two inspectors, and a permanent chairman. It would also have a permanent office, clerical support and the necessary statutory powers to ensure that its views and directives were enforced[8].

The interim Board of Control was established but the General Board of Commissioners of Lunacy never materialised. It was vehemently opposed by Lord Ashbourne, the lord chancellor for Ireland, who saw in it a diminution of his own judicial authority in regard to the supervision and protection of the insane[9]. But in any event changes in the Irish local government system were pending which would inevitably involve a review of the central and local administration of the asylums. When, eventually, the Local Government (Ireland) Act was enacted in 1898 it made fundamental changes in the system[10]. The Board of Control was abolished. The new county councils were assigned the role of operating the asylums, and the powers of the lord-lieutenant as to the appointment and removal of staff were transferred to them. Nevertheless, extensive powers of control remained vested in the lord-lieutenant, while the inspector's functions of visiting the asylums and inquiring into the care and treatment of the insane remained unaltered.

In none of its various manifestations did the central controlling board ever exercise any significant impact on lunacy policy. In so far as there was a dominant influence during the nineteenth century on the manner in which services for the insane evolved it may be said to have lain with the inspectors. It was an influence that ebbed and flowed depending on the indifference, enthusiasm and prejudices of individual inspectors and was, at times, hampered by their senility or ill-health.

Woodward and Palmer, already referred to, who became inspectors-general of prisons in 1822 were not doctors and showed no particular interest in the insane. Nevertheless by virtue of the fact that they were the only government officials with personal duties in relation to the supervision of the asylums they became the main advisers on lunacy matters to the lord-lieutenant. They were largely uninformed on the subject. Given their ignorance and indifference it was not surprising that the rules for the management of the asylums that the lord-lieutenant had been authorised to issue in 1821 did not appear until 1843 after Francis White had been made inspector of prisons on the death of Woodward[11].

The medical takeover

Two years earlier White, then surgeon to the Richmond asylum, had initiated a campaign to secure medical participation in the development of lunacy policy. He saw his appointment as an inspector of prisons as a first step in that direction. Now in a position to exercise some influence on the government he pressed for a lunacy inspectorate divorced from involvement with the prisons system except in so far as there were still insane persons detained in them. This was quickly conceded. An Act of 1845[12] provided for the creation of one or two posts of inspector of lunatics with the duty of inspecting and reporting on asylums and other institutions caring for lunatics. White became the first inspector, in January 1846, and was joined the following year by a second inspector, John Nugent, who had been travelling physician to Daniel O'Connell[13].

Subsequently, with White initially the main driving force, the two inspectors set out to consolidate the medical influence on the development and operation of the asylum system. Neither had any special experience or understanding of insanity to boost their authority but this was no disadvantage at a time when there was little scientifically based knowledge of either the nature or care of mental disorder. There was, however, general agreement among those involved with the problem that moral treatment with its emphasis on kindness and comfort was likely to give the best results. It was a broad easily understood and easily applied approach not yet complicated by the ideas of Freud or the language of psychoanalysis. But while it required little by way of expatiation or expert direction it was, in the inspectors' view, important that it evolve on medical principles. And here they were faced with obstacles in so far as the district lunatic asylums had already developed they had come almost entirely under lay control with doctors given only a secondary role.

In the absence of any significant medical influence the original concept of the district lunatic asylum system had been based largely on the notions of politicians and lay officials. Non-medical managers, sometimes referred to as 'moral superintendents', were placed in charge of each asylum as it opened. The dominant view of those in authority was, with some justification, that moral treatment was not substantially based on medical principles. In the circumstances there was no reason why an asylum should come under the exclusive direction of a doctor who probably lacked the potential for managing what was a more complex and costly type of institution than had hitherto existed. It was, however, accepted that there should be a physician on the staff appointed in a visiting capacity only.

There were no fixed qualifications for the posts of manager. The lord-lieutenant simply exercised his patronage on the basis of representations made to him. Samuel Wrigley, who became manager of the Richmond Asylum in 1832, had no professional qualifications of any sort nor any experience of dealing with the insane apart from a brief term of instruction in the Dublin House of Industry prior to taking up office[14]. The other managers holding office about this time would also appear to have undergone a period of induction in the same house of industry. Dr John Jacob of Maryborough, writing confidentially to the chief secretary in November 1833, alleged that most of them were related to each other, a situation that Jacob claimed was due to the excessive influence being exercised by one of the inspectors-general of prisons who himself was related to one of the managers[15].

The duties of the manager were daunting in their scope. His overall role was to superintend and regulate the whole asylum. He kept the minutes of the board and was responsible for maintaining a range of records and registers. He was required to supervise the staff and, if necessary, to discipline them by fine, suspension or dismissal, subject to the concurrence of the board.

He had daily to inspect each patient and 'make himself acquainted with every case'. He took charge of the instruments of restraint and recorded instances of their use but could not authorise the use of the shower-bath, a frequently used method of shock treatment, without the prior authority of the physician.

During meal times he was required to examine the conditions of the dining hall and the quality of the food; and when night came he had to walk through the dormitories and see that each patient was comfortably settled in his bed. He was also expected to be attentive to visitors and never to absent himself from the asylum at the same time as the matron. The matron, who was often the wife of the manager, was for her part required to supervise and report to the manager on the female patients and female staff. There was also a clerk/storekeeper whose role was a very subordinate one. While he kept the accounts, looked after the stores and took minutes at board meetings the primary responsibility for all these matters lay with the manager (and later medical superintendent) throughout the nineteenth century[16].

Long before White and Nugent became inspectors there was medical opposition to the placing of institutions under lay management. The most forthright and persistent of the critics was Dr John Jacob, already referred to, a governor of the Quaker institution, the Bloomfield Retreat, and proprietor of a private asylum in Maryborough. A pamphlet circulated by him to doctors in 1834 ridiculed the idea of anyone but a medical person being competent to apply moral treatment. He deplored the placing of a lunatic in the care of 'rude and illiterate keepers' whom he contrasted with 'the educated, intelligent philosopher and physician whom the eminent and the talented had been enlightening for the last two thousand years'[17]. There were other doctors, too, who campaigned in less abrasive terms than Jacob. Notable among them was Robert Stewart, the manager of Belfast Asylum, himself one of two managers with a medical background who, supported by his board of governors, urged the chief secretary in 1844 to confine management posts to medical men 'of high moral character and professional attainment'[18].

The doctors were less than fair to the lay managers who, in general, went about their work with considerable dedication. Some of them had condemned the more bizarre medical treatments such as the swing chair, the copious blood lettings and the plunging into cold baths. Thomas Jackson, for instance, lay manager of Armagh Asylum for a period, became widely known for his humane and enlightened methods[19].

But the doctors had much more influence than the lay managers. The asylum rules of 1843, of which White was almost certainly the begetter, were the first substantial step towards placing the asylums firmly within the province of medical control. As yet he was not in a position of sufficient influence to secure acceptance of the concept of medical management but the rules ensured that the actual treatment of the patients became exclusively a medical responsibility. They assigned to the visiting physician the direction of 'the moral and medical treatment' as well as the giving of advice to the governors as to when patients should be discharged. In furtherance of these duties he was required to attend the asylum on at least three days in the week or every day when there were more than 250 patients[20].

With the appointments of White and Nugent as first inspectors of lunatics the displacement of lay managers became inevitable. In their report for 1848 they were able to claim that the principle of appointing doctors to the manager posts had been recognised and reported that the visiting physician to Carlow District Asylum had been appointed manager there following the death of his lay predecessor. The process continued of replacement when the opportunity arose. All new asylums now had medical superintendents appointed *ab initio*. By 1853 nine of the then fourteen asylums were controlled by doctors. Six years later only one lay manager, Captain John Dobbs of Waterford, remained. All the physicians were required to reside in the asylums where they were provided with free apartments and food and an annual salary averaging about £300[21].

In order to influence the development of the asylums along

the lines they regarded as desirable the inspectors adopted a practice of attending in an informal manner the meetings of the various asylum boards. In April 1852 the governors of the Richmond Asylum suggested that they might be made *ex officio* members of that board as it would help to overcome the inconvenience of the occasional lack of a quorum. The lord-lieutenant agreed. The inspectors, taking advantage of the opportunity, then suggested that they might similarly be appointed to all other district asylum boards and this was done[22] . For a period they invariably took part in the meetings of the local boards, not in a muted way but involving themselves fully in discussions except to the extent that they did not vote on financial matters. Inevitably, perhaps, a certain amount of antipathy developed towards this practice among the local governors, who felt inhibited by the presence of the inspectors. The arrangement was dropped in 1861[23] .

Visiting physician versus medical superintendent

The transfer of the asylums from lay to medical management did not, as might be expected, lead to the termination of the office of visiting physician as had happened in the United Kingdom. The fact that there were now two doctors involved in decisions about the patients predictably proved fertile grounds for friction and led to considerable controversy among the doctors themselves.

It became clear from the beginning that those doctors who took up full-time salaried posts in the asylums were regarded by some of their profession as placing themselves in an inferior position. Their main critics came from among the visiting physicians who saw them as doctors of 'the hack class'[24] , professional mediocrities lacking not only the medical skills but the social distinction of the independent practitioner. Some of the doctors who had clamoured for medical control of the asylums now campaigned with even more vigour against the medical managers.

John Mollan, the visiting physician to the Richmond asylum, regarded medical managers as comparable to house surgeons, persons of junior status over whose views those of the visiting physician should prevail[25] . But the most virulent of the doctors opposed to giving the medical managers full discretion on medical matters was John Jacob who had been appointed visiting physician to Maryborough asylum. He contended that the role of the visiting physician was in effect that of the chief medical officer of the asylum; the resident medical superintendent should obey his orders and 'not be in a position to raise difficulties'[26] . Jacob pushed the issue to extremes with Burton, the medical superintendent of the Maryborough institution. The patients, it appears, supported Burton. When Jacob visited the asylum he had to be protected from them by a guard of attendants, obscene rhymes were composed about him, and on one occasion he was struck by a stone thrown by a female patient. Eventually it became necessary in 1861 to have a five day public enquiry carried out in the asylum which culminated in Burton being transferred to another asylum and Jacob reprimanded for lack of 'forbearance and consideration for the feelings of those associated with him'[27] .

The major influence for retaining the visiting physician posts was exerted by the lunacy inspectors. When the commissioners established in 1856 to investigate the general operation of the lunacy services heard evidence from Francis White he left them in no doubt as to his view. The treatment of asylum patients should be carried out in consultation with a visiting physician so 'as not to leave entirely the whole medical management to a man who probably never goes outside the asylum'[28] . When the commissioners made their recommendations they were divided on the subject. The lay majority favoured giving the resident medical physician responsibility for the care of the physical and mental illness of the patient, the role of the visiting physician to be confined to cases in which the former required consultation[29] . But one of the commissioners Dr Dominic Corrigan, distinguished and influential president of the Royal College of Physicians of Ireland, disagreed. His attitude represented that of the then medical establishment. Implicitly critical of the quality of the asylum doctors, he was concerned about placing treatment under the 'uncontrolled management' of one person. The involvement of the visiting physician would, he suggested, be welcomed by the friends of patients and lessen their reluctance to have them admitted to the asylum[30] .

During 1861 the chief secretary, Sir Robert Peel, heard view and counter-view from separate deputations representing the visiting physicians and the resident superintendents. The latter were by now organised with their British counterparts. The Association of Medical Officers of Asylums and Hospitals for the Insane, established in 1841, was publishing its own clinical journal and was determined on securing recognition for the asylum doctors as experts in the care of insanity. When eventually in 1862 the Irish Privy Council agreed to revised rules for the management of the asylums the changes represented some gain for the resident physicians but did not remove the irritant of the visiting physician[31] . The resident doctors were given clear responsibility for the mental and general medical treatment of the patients subject to consultation with the physicians in difficult cases. But both doctors had to examine the mental condition of patients prior to discharge and to sign the necessary certificate. Furthermore the inspectors of lunacy were empowered, if they considered it desirable, to require the visiting physician to attend daily at the asylum and to report to them on any matters about which the inspectors required information.

Inferentially this last requirement allowed the visiting physician to be used as a spy for the inspectors. While it was seen as such there is no evidence that it was used to any extent. But it certainly underlined the lack of confidence by the central administration in the hospital managers. Francis White had retired as inspector in 1857 following injuries received in a train accident[32] . He was succeeded by George Hatchell, and White's former colleague, John Nugent, a man of strong views, now became the dominant figure in the lunacy office and was to remain so for over thirty years. The rules of 1862 reflected his attitude towards the resident superintendents. He remained consistently of the view that they were men of limited ability and that it was in the interests of the inmates and the public that they should have the assistance of visiting physicians whether they liked it or not[33]. He was prepared to maintain this view and to support troublesome visiting physicians even when, as described later, it led to a breakdown in the proper administration of the Central Criminal Lunatic Asylum in Dundrum.

Nevertheless, most of the late nineteenth century visiting and resident doctors worked agreeably together despite the fact that the divided medical responsibility undoubtedly diminished the professional standing of the resident manager. The lunacy office had turned the asylum superintendent into the drudge of Irish medicine. His medical skills were disparaged while at the same time any possibility that he might develop those skills and give more time to medical practice was effectively ruled out by the huge burden of administrative duties of a non-medical nature which he was required to carry out. As asylums became overcrowded and costs soared he had to face irate boards of governors concerned about the demands on public funds. Socially and politically he had none of the influence of the visiting physician who often led the life of a country gentleman supported by the patronage of the landlords and office-holders of the establishment. An English commentator on the Irish asylums system wrote in 1891:

> . . . in most places the visiting physicianship is simply an item among the small appointments that go to aid the practitioner of a country town. If the board are friendly the post can be transferred along with the other perquisities of a practice, or may even be hereditary[34].

The asylum rules of 1862 were reviewed on various occasions during the subsequent thirty years but both posts remained with little change in their roles[35]. But with the passage of time there were developments that strengthened the case for the independence of the resident superintendent. Towards the end of the century the concept of the specialist doctor had clearly emerged in various areas of medicine, including the treatment of the insane. Furthermore, a considerable volume of scientific speculation and postulation had developed about the origins and therapy of insanity. The argument that a general practitioner should have the key professional role in the conduct of an asylum was becoming increasingly untenable. While change was inevitable it was accelerated by disputes concerning the Central Criminal Lunatic Asylum at Dundrum that not only highlighted the divisive potential of visiting physician posts but revealed the shortcomings of the lunacy inspectors themselves.

Trouble in Dundrum

The law had placed the regulation of the Dundrum asylum and the appointment of its staff under the direct control of the lord-lieutenant. In practice it was directed by the two inspectors of lunacy operating from their small office within the headquarters of the chief secretary in Dublin Castle. Since they were doctors committed to a policy of distancing the care of the insane from its long-time association with the prison system the inspectors were determined to organise the Dundrum asylum on the same basis as a district asylum and to submerge as far as they could the prison elements of its role. It was, in their view, primarily an institution for insane persons who should be treated as patients and not as criminals.

Those concerned with the administration of the criminal law thought otherwise. The asylum was above all a prison concerned with punishment rather than care and it should be managed and organised on that basis. Nugent, summarised the issue:

> The subject at issue resolves itself into the simple question whether an individual mentally affected who may have broken the law while so affected or, after a criminal act, becomes insane, is to be regarded and subsequently treated more as a lunatic or a criminal. I contend that . . . because an aberration of mind in

the first case condones the offence however serious
and in the second case entails a condonation where
the malady exists (the inmate) should be therefore
excluded from the category of an ordinary prisoner
undergoing a punishment for guilt[36] .

For a considerable period Nugent's view prevailed. As senior
inspector he effectively ran the asylum insisting always that
the medical governor should not be given too much authority
otherwise the supervision by the lunacy department would be
reduced 'to a mere shadow'[37] . The inmates were subjected
to the same regimen as those in ordinary district asylums; their
'merely . . . legal criminality' was ignored but in view of the
obligation to ensure their secure custody there was a slightly
higher proportion of attendants than in other asylums[38] .

But there were in the arrangements for the administration
of the asylum elements of inevitable conflict. The paramountcy
of Nugent and his fellow inspector, Hatchell, reduced the
status and the authority of the governor. It was further
weakened by the fact that the asylum continued to have a
visiting physician so that in practice there was a tripartite
direction that eventually led to continuing dispute between
the parties and to a series of special committees of enquiry
in the period 1882-1891. The main clashes occurred between
Dr Isaac Ashe, a well-intentioned liberal-minded governor,
and Dr John Hughes, the visiting physician, who frequently
interfered with Ashe's management of patients and issued
countermanding directions to the staff. Nugent also meddled
in the day-to-day affairs of the asylum and invariably supported Hughes.

Faced with continuing complaints about the operation of
the asylum, including some from Dr McCabe, the Catholic
archbishop of Dublin, the lord-lieutenant established a committee of enquiry in 1881[39] . It examined various allegations
ranging from the mistreatment of patients to such trivia as
the consumption of a quart of cream daily by Dr Ashe and
his family when his conditions of appointment entitled him
to draw only a pint from the asylum's farm. The enquiry

confirmed some instances of neglect and mistreatment. These included the case of a troublesome female patient kept in a strait-jacket for an unbroken period of eight months. There was evidence that another patient named Mahoney, self-titled Cneius Pompeius, Magnus the Great, had been confined in a cell for four days for refusing to take off his hat when 'God Save the Queen' was played at a dance in the asylum.

Dancing itself was also the cause of complaint and investigation. The governor, Ashe, had arranged a weekly dance for the inmates 'at which waltzing and polkas were most favoured'. The visiting physician forbade it. He had the support of Nugent who was aghast at the idea of homicidal maniacs of both sexes dancing together in an 'exhibition (that) could not be of a very edifying character'. The Catholic chaplain shared their opposition; he made it clear that he 'objected altogether to dancing in every class of life'.

Incongruously, Nugent, whose own supervision of the asylum was implicitly an issue, had been made chairman of the enquiry. The other two members, Dr Arthur Mitchell, commissioner of lunacy in Scotland and W.R. Holmes, treasury remembrancer in Ireland, ignored him and wrote their own report. They recommended that the supreme authority for the management of the asylum be vested in the governor and that the roles of the inspectors and the visiting physician be reduced. Nugent protested indignantly in a separate submission to the lord-lieutenant.

After a long delay a few new minor rules were issued about the daily operation of the asylum such as the appropriate rations of milk for the patients and staff[40]. The main recommendations made by Mitchell and Holmes were ignored. No changes were made in the administration of the institution nor in the powers of the inspectorate. It was abundantly clear that as far as Dublin Castle was concerned Nugent ruled the roost in regard to the lunatic asylums. Given the dramatic political backdrop of the period it would have been surprising if the affairs of the lunacy office were to engender any interest elsewhere in the Irish administration. The demands for agrarian reform and home rule and the preoccupation of government and people alike with Parnell and his policies made narrow social issues like that of the administration of the lunacy services a matter of little significance. Questions of this sort were best left to those public officials who were being paid to look after them, even if their own stewardship was being questioned.

Hughes, the visiting physician, died during 1882 and was replaced by Dr C.J. Nixon with whom Ashe, the governor, appeared to develop a happier relationship[41]. But the basic weakness in the administration arising from its tripartite nature remained. Complaints continued to be made. More patients than usual were escaping owing, it was said, to the defects in the management of the asylum. Eventually in 1885 the lord-lieutenant asked Mitchell and Holmes to carry out another enquiry this time without the involvement of Nugent.

When they reported they were, as they had been previously, highly critical of the administration of the asylum and satisfied that the close personal involvement of the inspectors was leading 'to a conflict of jurisdiction and to innefficiency[42]. The report recommended that the institution be placed under the control of the General Prisons Board with the inspectors of lunacy merely having a visiting and reporting role. The enquirers conceded that when the asylum was originally provided for in 1845 it was:

> ... no doubt called an asylum as an outcome of views regarding the relations of insanity to crime which were earnestly advocated and were in the ascendent for some years. ...

Now, they argued, there was a different view. The primary function of such an institution was seen as that of a prison for the safe custody of persons lodged there as prisoners whether or not they were also lunatics.

Again Nugent in a memorandum to under-secretary Sir Robert Hamilton contested the findings of the inquiry, particularly the recommendation that the institution be regarded as a prison rather than an asylum[43]. It was, he wrote, 'a fallacious theory'; the institution was fundamentally an asylum and the recommendation should be rejected. Again he was successful in preventing change and the report was ignored.

A few years later some of the main personalities left the scene and a fresh and more objective evaluation of the Dundrum asylum and the broader issues raised by it in regard to the inspectors and visiting physician became possible. Hatchell died during 1889. Nugent, after forty-three years service, retired with a knighthood, the inevitable award for any senior official whose career had been bland and time-serving. 'Poor goody Dr Ashe', as he was described privately by Arthur Mitchell, died in 1890[44]. In 1891 the lord-lieutenant appointed yet another committee of enquiry into the affairs of the asylum. The four-man committee included the two new inspectors of lunacy, Dr George Plunkett O'Farrell and Dr E. Maziere Courtenay. They were younger and more energetic men than their predecessors and more favourably disposed towards asylum doctors. O'Farrell had previously been a medical inspector of the Local Government Board; Courtenay was formerly medical superintendent of Limerick asylum and had earlier been responsible for founding the Irish branch of the Medico-Psychological Association[45].

There was unanimity in their findings and recommen-dations[46]. The members found in the asylum 'an all pervading confusion and disorder in association with the disloyalty and faithlessness of the attendants of whom the governor states that few are really trustworthy'. The committee had no doubt that the low level of discipline had been aggravated by the 'weakness and confusion' caused by the participation of the inspectors in the administration of the asylum. It had not been helped either by the existence of the office of visiting physician which was in itself 'a prejudicial disturbance in the balance of authority'. The committee was satisfied that the proper administration of the Dundrum asylum could only be restored by limiting the role of the inspectors to a purely inspectorial one and by abolishing the office of visiting physician. Once again it was recommended that the institution be transferred to the immediate supervision and control of the General Prisons Board. The findings were considerably strengthened when the government committee looking at broader aspects of Irish lunacy policy made similar recommendations in 1891[47].

While no action was taken about the responsibility for Dundrum asylum the government acted quickly in regard to the visiting physicians. An order made by the lord-lieutenant in December 1891 declared that henceforth when a vacancy in the office of visiting physician occurred in any district asylum the post was to be abolished. Where a post was terminated it was replaced by that of an assistant medical officer[48]. There was a predictable outcry by the medical establishment, including the Council of the Royal College of Surgeons in Ireland, who in newspaper correspondence continued to portray the asylum superintendents as poorly qualified doctors motivated by 'personal ambition and love of power'. There were, too, insinuations that they wished to conceal their maltreatment of patients[49]. These were grossly unfair criticisms which, by creating an unfavourable image of asylum care, did nothing to advance the interests of the insane.

The governors

From the beginning of the system responsibility for the local government of the district lunatic asylums was given to boards of governors appointed by the lord-lieutenant[50]. Most of the governors were drawn from the local ascendency and many of them also served as grand jurors or held other public offices. They were predominantly Protestant, the few Catholics usually being confined to the local bishop and to landed gentry of the 'Castle Catholic' variety untainted by nationalist inclinations. The records suggest that few of them took any real humanitarian interest in the asylums. As they saw it, their appointments came as a due and expected recognition of their status and power, a confirmation of their membership of the ruling *élite* rather than the assignment of a duty to be performed.

From their point-of-view an important consideration was that being an asylum governor extended the range of patronage available to them. It was a patronage that applied both to the admission of patients and to the filling of jobs. The normal form of admission of patients involved the presentation of a medical certificate of insanity and a declaration of poverty on behalf of the next-of-kin. From among the applicants the governors selected the cases to fill the available vacancies although many families ensured admission by getting a judicial direction that the patient was dangerous[51]. The posts of visiting physician and all subordinate jobs in the asylum were filled by the governors; the lord-lieutenant retained to himself the appointment of the managers, the later resident medical superintendents and, for a period, the matrons[52]. The governors jealously guarded their own powers. Some who were members of parliament protested strongly during 1856 when a parliamentary committee was discussing legislative proposals to give clearer authority to the lord-lieutenant in regard to asylum appointments. Isaac Butt, then a governor of the Cork asylum, asserted vehemently that he 'would not be the cats-paw of the lord-lieutenant or a jobbing chief secretary' and promised that if the proposals were enacted he would never again enter Cork asylum as a governor. There was, too, indignant opposition from Captain Magan, a governor of Mullingar asylum, who pointed to the matron in Mullingar as an example of the poor quality of the lord-lieutenant's appointments and claimed that she 'had long been considered the nuisance of the establishment'[53].

Similar resentment emerged when there was any indication of the weakening of the governors' authority in regard to the admission of patients. The board of Carlow asylum protested to the chief secretary during 1844 that the power given to medical officers to admit patients in cases of urgency was 'setting aside the authority of a body of gentlemen who, at great personal inconvenience, give up their time gratuitously to the public'[54].

There was, in fact, no evidence of governors in general putting themselves to inconvenience although the central administration for a considerable period maintained the myth that their contribution was a valuable one. Because of the power they commanded they were treated with great deference by the inspectors of lunacy and often referred to patronisingly by them. The inspectors believed that 'gentlemen of education, rank and position offered the best guarantee of efficient management'[55]. Yet many of them rarely or never visited the asylum or attended the monthly meeting of the board. Despite the large numbers (sometimes as many as forty-five) of governors appointed to boards, it was at times impossible to secure the required quorum of three for a meeting. It was often necessary following a meeting for a messenger to ride as many as thirty miles in order to get the signature of an additional member to allow the accounts to be approved[56]. The disinterest applied not only to meetings but to conditions in the asylums. 'It is too much the habit with country gentlemen to gloss over these things' chided Dr White timorously in 1843, when he found primitive conditions in Cork asylum which some of the governors had never seen for themselves[57].

But over the next fifty years all the asylums continued to be in the charge of indifferent governors. In 1858 a report of a government commission of enquiry recommended that in future two thirds of the asylum governors should be appointed by the local grand juries[58]. Influenced by the recommendations, Lord Naas, the Irish chief secretary, introduced a bill under which asylum visitors would be appointed by the local grand jury to exercise the powers of the governors hitherto appointed by the lord-lieutenant. It was presented as a measure aimed at decentralising authority and emphasising local responsibility. But it could hardly be described as a gesture towards the more democratic government of the asylums; the grand juries themselves were ascendency and sectarian in character and unlikely to appoint visitors markedly different from the chosen *élite* of the lord-lieutenant. In any event the bill was dropped with a change of government in June 1859[59].

During 1871 nineteen of the thirty-five governors in Belfast failed to attend a single meeting. In Mullingar during the same year twenty-seven of the forty-six members had a similar record and twelve of the remainder attended only once or twice in the year[60]. The general rules for the regulation of the asylums required two or more governors to inspect each asylum once a month. In 1872 according to the inspectors of lunacy no inspections were carried out in some asylums and in others they 'were very irregularly performed'[61]. Yet, in general, the central lunacy administration was prepared to cast a blind eye on the inactivity of the governors. In 1876 the inspectors reported that the attendance of governors in most asylums was 'full and regular' when tables appended to the same report clearly showed that this was not so[62]. Seven years later there was no change in the situation. The average attendance at board meetings in Maryborough and Ennis was three, a not untypical situation[63]. It was not until 1888 against a background of growing demands for a democratic system of local government that the lord-lieutenant removed many of the governors who, from age or indifference, were then inactive. But as yet there was little recognition of the majority population. The replacements were a further selection of 'the gentry and educated body of society'[64]. But with the coming of the county council system change was only a decade away.

Heredity, Moral Weakness
or Tea

As the nineteenth century progressed the mounting toll of insanity was, for those in authority, an alarming one as much for its financial as for its social implications. It was not an uniquely Irish problem although by the end of the century it had become evident that Ireland was an extreme example. In other western countries, too, the introduction of special provisions for the insane had set off an unexpected demand which gave rise to considerable speculation about the causes of insanity and its growing incidence.

A number of themes dominate the professional literature of the period. Insanity, some argued, was an inherited factor acquired from one's ancestors in the same way as wealth or social standing. Others saw it as largely a manifestation of moral weakness, the outcome of dissipation and self-indulgence. The more general view was that various factors were involved and that civil disturbance and the growing complexity of nineteenth century society were aggravating influences. But none could find a definable line of demarcation between madness and normality. Scull has commented:

> The implications of this situation were profound. Beyond the initial hard core of easily recognisable behavioural and/or mental disturbance, the boundary between the normal and the pathological was left extraordinarily vague and indeterminate. In consequence insanity was such an amorphous all-embracing concept

that the range of behaviour it could be stretched to encompass was almost infinite[1].

The introduction of a system of large institutions for such a vaguely defined condition had particular implications for Ireland. It was not, of course, the only national network of institutions. As already described the poor law of 1838 had provided the workhouses and they were readily availed of during the 1840s when, in conditions of abject famine, they offered for many the only prospect of survival. But the poor law system was such that it was devised to deter and to shame. It was successful in doing so. By the time the great famine had passed and the survivors of the catastrophe had resumed their normal pattern of life the local poorhouse had come to be regarded as a place of last resort, resented and shunned by every self-respecting person.

Yet pauperism remained high and living standards among the great bulk of the population, particularly those in rural areas, continued to be harsh even at the best of times. But while the burden of having a member who was chronically ill or infirm intensified the hardships of many a family, relatively few would have contemplated resort to the poor law system. The lunatic asylum, however, offered a less objectionable alternative. It was caring in its conception; it cost nothing, and it had less deterring conditions than the workhouse. While it, too, was often regarded as imposing a stigma on the family it never, at any time, appears to have attracted the detestation directed at the latter. Many took advantage of the comparative ease with which persons could be accepted as insane and admitted to the asylum to rid themselves of relatives and friends who were a burden or a nuisance. By the 1870s the inspectors were complaining about the widespread tendency to send unsuitable patients to the asylums:

> ... if there be any excuse whatever for doing so, no matter how hopeless or indefinite the symptoms of the disease may be; the bed-ridden, aged, the infirm alike, and even children when troublesome, noisy, difficult of control or idiotic are constantly drafted

off to district asylums as dangerous. What is even still worse, it occasionally happens that persons in a state of extreme physical exhaustion or actual dying, are committed upon the strength of magisterial warrants, females alike with males[2].

But despite this abuse of the asylum system the great majority of admissions had at least some manifestation of insanity if one accepts as reasonably honest the statistical tables returned annually by the asylum authorities. Throughout most of the latter half of the century the main classifications used for the illness of patients were mania, monomania, dementia, melancholia, imbecility and epilepsy, and idiocy. Later mania and monomania were integrated and general paralysis of the insane was added[3]. Since some of these classifications were vague in concept and with little scientific basis there could not have been any real uniformity of diagnosis in the asylums.

The probable causes of illness were classified under two broad headings – moral and physical. The moral causes included poverty, grief, love affairs, domestic quarrels, mental anxiety and religious excitement. There were obviously other harmful excitements. In 1855, at the time of the Crimean War, the inspectors noted the number of military men in the private asylums when 'the warlike spirit of the country was at its highest point'[4]. Since the private asylums maintained only those in a position to pay, the individuals concerned were almost certainly of the officer class and members of ascendency families. While they may have been driven mad by military fervour it also seems possible that they had made a conscious choice of an asylum environment to the battlefields of Sebastopol. In general, however, women tended to be more vulnerable than men to insanity of moral origins. The inspectors explained that this was due to the fact that because they were 'corporeally weaker and weaker in reasoning power their susceptibilities are stronger and more acute'[5]. Nevertheless the annual reports of the inspectors show that overall there was a preponderance of males in the asylums of the Victorian period. This has continued to be so.

The physical causes included hereditary influences, intemperance, sun-stroke, venereal disease and masturbation. The latter was 'a fruitful source of insanity' wrote Dr Edward O'Neill of Limerick District Asylum in 1893[6]. Dr O'Neill's view was a fairly widely held one. In Ireland asylum statistics would suggest that insanity associated with masturbation was regarded as exclusively a male hazard. In Victorian Britain it was often related to females as well. Female madness was considered to have a strong association with various aspects of female sexuality. The life cycle of a woman was seen as bedevilled with biological crises such as nymphomania, puerperal mania and ovarian madness. Isaac Baker Brown, a prominent London gynaecologist, offered preventive procedures in his large private clinic where he practised sexual surgery, including clitorectomy, before being expelled from the Obstetrical Society of London towards the end of the 1860s[7].

Heredity

In regard to asylum admissions for which a specific cause of illness was assigned the hereditary factor was by far the largest. By the 1890s the consensus everywhere was that insanity was mainly hereditary in origin. Burdett summarised the prevailing opinion in 1891[8]. He wrote:

> Much concerning insanity is doubtful, and few things there are believed in by one physician which will not be flatly denied by another; but one thing is never doubted, and that is the terribly hereditary nature of insanity.

It was a view that had almost universal support among Irish doctors. In 1894 the inspectors of lunacy believed that it was the main source of insanity in Ireland. It was a belief shared by most of the asylum superintendents[9]. Dr E.E. Moore of Letterkenny asylum considered heredity to be the predisposing cause of insanity in seventy per cent of admissions to his asylum. Consanguineous marriages were aggravating the hazard according to some superintendents. Dr W.H. Garner reported on local circumstances that gave rise to many such marriages in Tipperary. The Dwyers, Mahers, Ryans and O'Briens were faction fighting families who sometimes met in violent feud at fairs and markets. These families constituted a large segment of the Tipperary population and since marriage between them was taboo they tended to marry within their own families. Garner claimed that a considerable element of the then patient population in Clonmel asylum were the offspring of such marriages.

On the other hand Dr Connolly Norman, of the Richmond asylum, who was probably the most enlightened and progressive Irish asylum doctor of the period, was not convinced that there was sufficient evidence to justify giving so much weight to the heredity theory. But he had few supporters. The widespread acceptance by doctors and general public alike that some families were transmitters of insanity maintained and strengthened public prejudice. The stigma associated with insanity grew in strength. But it was not always a deterrent to marriage into an afflicted family. A Donegal priest wrote 'if there be money in the question, or a farm, insanity would not be considered'[10].

Tea and alcohol

Some of the asylum superintendents believed that a major influence on Irish insanity lay in poor nutrition standards. Tea was seen as a particular hazard; many persons had developed the habit of drinking large quantities of it after it had been left 'stewing' at length. Tea and bread had become the main sustenance for most poorer families in substitution for the former dietary of porridge, milk and potatoes. Dr G.W. Hatchell (son of one of the inspectors), who was in charge of Castlebar District Asylum, complained in 1893 that the spread of the tea-drinking habit was being encouraged by travelling tea salesmen who drove in carts throughout the countryside. Dr William Graham of Armagh gave a similar account of pedlars 'seated in gay croydons heavily laden with Indian teas which they sell to poor people at an exorbitant profit'. And about the same time Dr E.E. Moore of Letterkenny wrote 'this tea-drinking is becoming a curse, and the people are developing a craving for tea just as great as that which a drunkard has for alcohol . . .'[11].

Whatever about the consumption of tea and its harmful effects there was certainly a craving for alcohol, although excessive drinking declined from the mid-century onwards. Illicit stills proliferated in the early decades of the century. Wakefield wrote ' . . . they are erected in the kitchens of baronets and in the stables of clergymen'[12]. For many, drinking became the only escape from the dire realities of the period; huge quantities of home-distilled whiskey were consumed particularly in rural areas. However, with the more effective application of the excise laws and under the influence of Father Theobald Mathew, the 'apostle of temperance', there was a continuing decline in the consumption of spirits from the 1840s onwards[13]. Excessive drinking remained, however, one of the principal causes of admission to both the district and private lunatic asylums. In 1857 the inspectors reported that 'cases of moral madness originating in drink and dissipation' were being frequently admitted to the private asylums[14].

It is of interest, however, that while intemperance was always one of the main causes of admission to the district lunatic asylums these admissions represented only a relatively small proportion of the total. About seven per cent of all patients in these asylums at the end of March 1861 had been admitted for that reason. During 1893 about nine per cent of admissions were due to excessive drinking. Various medical superintendents reported during the following years that alcoholism was not a serious cause of admission. Dr Connolly Norman noted 'people drink less than they used to'[15]. Nevertheless an upward trend in asylum admissions from alcoholism was becoming evident and during the decade prior to 1906 about fifteen per cent of all admissions were due to that cause[16]. It contrasts with the present pattern of admissions to Irish psychiatric hospitals; in 1982 over twenty-five per cent of all admissions were related to alcoholism[17].

While the explanation for the big increase in the number of alcoholics seeking care in modern times probably lies to a large extent in the greater consumption of alcohol another important factor must be considered in comparing past and present patterns. The perception of alcoholism, particularly its relevance to treatment in an asylum for the insane, was somewhat different in Victorian times. The notion that alcoholism was a disease became popular with some American and British physicians during the late nineteenth century and Maudsley discussed 'alcoholic insanity' in 1879[18]. But the contemporary returns of Irish asylum superintendents suggest that the alcoholic was admitted only when his excessive drinking was believed to be the 'exciting' cause of insane ideas or actions. Chronic heavy drinking without other irrational behaviour was not yet generally seen as having a connection with mental disturbance. The notion of alcoholism as an addiction and of addiction being in itself a mental abnormality had not yet clearly emerged. Drunkenness in public was regarded as a petty crime and was often punished by imprisonment. No specific provisions existed for the therapy of the drunkard who was widely seen to be the victim of his own self-indulgence and not of disease. A pamphleteer wrote in 1882 'every human soul is worth saving but . . . if a choice is to be made, drunkards are about the last class to be taken hold of'[19]. It was the common view.

Where concern existed for the drunkard it was seen in terms of moral reform rather than cure and was mainly manifested through the exhortations of temperance movements, individual clergymen, and lay evangelists. But towards the end of the century there was a view that the reform of the inveterate non-criminal drunkard required a more aggressive approach involving some form of institutional care.

Largely as a result of a campaign undertaken by Sir Charles Cameron, this view eventually led to a series of special statutes beginning with the Habitual Drunkards Act, 1879[20]. The new provisions applied to Britain and Ireland and related to the drunkard not considered insane who was a danger to himself or others or incapable of managing his affairs. Their novel and distinctive feature was that they offered to the habitual drunkard the possibility of having himself voluntarily locked away for a period not exceeding twelve months. Confinement was to be in a 'retreat', a house licensed for that purpose by the local authority.

The measures when first discussed in parliament were generally welcomed but some members saw them as a threat to the liberty of the individual. The view was expressed that it was better to be 'free than sober'[21]. In order to meet these criticisms and reduce the possibility of abuse, the statutory safeguards subsequently written into the legislation were so fulsome that not only was abuse made difficult but formidable obstacles were placed in the way of confining anyone. If a drunkard decided to seek self-immurement he had to make a written application accompanied by a statutory declaration from two persons asserting that he was a habitual drunkard. Furthermore two justices of the peace had then not only to attest his signature but also themselves to be satisfied that he was a drunkard[22].

The response to the new legislation in Ireland, as in Britain, was minimal. One retreat was established: The Lodge opened by the Irish Women's Temperance Union in Belfast in 1902. Restricted to female patients, it admitted during the period, 1902-16 an annual average of only thirteen patients[23]. The original legislation was amended in 1898, and the additional measures provided for inebriate reformatories, a further new type of institution in which habitual drunkards guilty of crime might be detained for up to three years[24]. The reformatories could be operated by the government or by licensed individuals but in this regard, too, there was little response. Ennis jail was renovated and re-opened as a state reformatory in 1899; the small number of inebriates there were occasionally to be seen walking, under escort, outside its walls[25]. Two small religious controlled licensed reformatories were opened in Waterford (1906) and Wexford (1910) but both had closed down by 1920[26]. None of these new institutions had ever aroused any real interest and in so far as excessive drinkers were concerned the lunatic asylums continued, increasingly, to accept the burden of their care.

Religious fervour

Religious fervour was seen during the nineteenth century as the origin of some of the more extreme instances of abnormal mental behaviour. Burdett in his account in 1891 of lunatic asylums throughout the world expressed a view commonly held by those who were not themselves closely involved in religious affairs:

> Religion has always a powerful effect upon the insane and its effect is most commonly not for good, while religious mania is probably the most hopeless form of insanity[27].

Casting doubts on any aspect of the role of religion was, however, a hazardous matter in nineteenth century Ireland. For the government it was an especially sensitive issue; anxious to placate and win the support of the Catholic population it was determined from early in the century to distance itself from the religious proselytism previously associated with public institutions. For that reason it was necessary that the new lunatic asylums and workhouses should not only be seen to be utterly impartial in religious matters but that their inmates should be facilitated in every way in the practice of their religion. This policy necessarily involved the appointment of chaplains.

Given the belief that 'religious excitement' could be harmful there was some concern that the asylum chaplains might have a disturbing influence on patients. It was not helped by the fact that a disproportionate number of clergymen and other religious were themselves to be found among the insane inmates. This created some embarrassment for the inspectors but they were quick to point out that it would be 'a mistake to assume that the delusions of the individuals in question turn on purely divine or metaphysical points; they almost invariably refer to much more sublunary objects'[28].

In any event, during the 1850s, the two inspectors, Nugent and White, were determined to secure the implementation of government policy in regard to chaplains. They occasionally visited the asylums during religious service and questioned both patients and attendants about the effects of the ministrations of the clergymen. They reported:

> ... we cannot arrive at any other conclusion than that the regular visitations of chaplains, and the due performance of divine worship, should not be denied to the inmates of public institutions for the insane; for apart from other and higher considerations, the soothing influence of religion as tending to the establishment of a self-control however temporary in its nature, cannot but be valuable in a curative point of view ... [29].

Thereafter the firm policy of the central lunacy office was one of insistence that the appointment of chaplains was in the best interests of the patients.

There were, however, rebellious boards of governors who held a different view about the beneficial influence of chaplains and stuck to it. In Clonmel, Armagh and Belfast no chaplains were appointed[30]. The Belfast governors were particularly adamant. Under pressure from the government to change their stance they wrote to the lord-lieutenant in December 1851 vehemently defending their decision. They quoted various medical opinions rejecting the view that religious services had a favourable effect on the minds of the insane and alleged that 'it is one of the monomanias of the present day the extremes to which the exercise of religion is carried on professionally in our lunatic asylums'. And they suggested that a situation which involved three or four different chaplains each conducting a separate Sunday service under the same roof was 'calculated to cause no small excitement even among the sane'.

The government persisted in its determination to bring the Belfast governors to heel. In 1853 it appointed chaplains of its own to the asylum but the governors refused to admit them. Even when the government offered to pay their salaries the board still refused to accept the appointments. Eventually, taking the only other course available it sought a mandamus to the board from the courts. It was refused. After this defeat the government gave up trying. Eventually in 1870 over forty years after the opening of the asylum the Belfast governors admitted three chaplains, a Catholic, a Protestant and a Presbyterian, following assurances given by the appointees that they would do nothing to disturb the harmony of the asylum[31]. The Armagh and the Clonmel disputes had by then also been settled.

In refusing for so long to admit chaplains the Belfast governors were probably far more perspicacious than the government. While the latter's primary concern was to insist on the universal acceptance of a basic principle of religious policy, the Belfast governors had to face the reality that the area they served was in a frequent state of religious ferment. Understandably they did not wish to import into their asylum either the religious hysteria or the religious antagonisms so much a feature of Ulster life. During the period of the dispute a revivalist campaign carried on in various parts of Ulster in 1859 provided ample evidence of the extent to which some minds could be disturbed by frenzied religious activity.

Reverend W. Gibson, a former moderator of the Presbyterian Church, had, with some other preachers, studied the methods of American revivalism and introduced them to Ulster and to Belfast in particular[32]. Their preaching was intense and phrenetic, concentrating on the enormity of sin and the certainty of damnation for the sinner. 'Hell, hell is the one cry; physical and metaphysical hell' wrote one Protestant clergyman who had watched the revivalists in action. The preachers, sometimes as young as twelve years of age, often identified the damned among their listeners. 'Your case is as bad as hell can make it' said one pointing to a young girl who then collapsed[33].

The frenzy caused by the movement reached its height in Belfast in July 1859. Crowds gathered at street corners in the working class areas to hear the preachers. From time to time jaunting cars were to be seen moving through the streets conveying home the casualties of the preaching, usually young girls, supported in the arms of friends, sometimes in a swoon, sometimes screaming and crying hysterically. On occasion miraculous apparitions were claimed. Two Presbyterian clergymen who conducted a prayer meeting at Drum, County Monaghan, asserted that at least three hundred of those present had seen God descending from a black cloud[34].

There was no doubt about the temporary impact the campaign had on the pattern of insanity in the Ulster counties. A Belfast clergyman claimed that it had given rise to at least fifty cases in his own immediate area. The medical superintendent of Omagh asylum reported the admission of twenty-six cases for which the movement was 'the exciting cause'; with one exception all had a predisposition to insanity. One of these patients wished to dance naked 'before the Ark' and another had tried to pluck out her eyes because they were offending members. The inspectors of lunacy in their annual report referred to the influence of the revivalist preachers and noted that in one district it had caused more cases of insanity within a few months than had taken place in the whole preceding year[35].

It was, however, a passing phenomenon. Intense religious agitation in Ireland during the nineteenth century had two distinctive elements. There was, in the first instance, the wider and longer sustained activities outside of Ulster of well-endowed Protestant missionary societies determined to save Irish Catholics from the errors of popery. This lasted from the early years of the century until the 1860s when, disappointed by the fruits of their harvest, the societies ran out of steam and their labours rapidly diminished[36]. The Ulster campaign was briefer and different in character. In this instance Presbyterian preachers set out to increase the religious solidity of their flock threatened, as they saw it, not only by an evil world but by the mass of intransigent papistry by which it was surrounded. However, by the end of the 1860s the religious environment in general had become less intense and, as far as insanity was concerned, the harmful influence of messianic zealots had become of little consequence.

Emigration and insanity

The consequences of mass-emigration during this period also had implications in regard to the pattern of Irish insanity. As information became available about the impact of nineteenth century immigrants on their adopted countries it provided indications that the Irish who left home during the famine and post-famine decades were more susceptible to insanity than immigrants of other racial origins. Even by the mid-century there was evidence of Irish vulnerability.

During the 1840s and 1850s, as the stream of Irish migrants flowed into the United States and settled mainly along the north eastern coast the demands for asylum accommodation increased in these areas. The opening of new institutions in the State of Massachusetts and the municipality of Boston reflected this unwelcome aspect of the impact of the Irish immigrant. Before the 1840s the provisions in that region for the insane had been relatively small; with the arrival of large numbers of Irish people Massachusetts found it necessary to build two new asylums and a further one was erected by the Boston authorities. Their first inmates were largely Irish labourers[37].

Over the next half century the evidence of the Irish emigrants' susceptibility to insanity grew. By 1900 53.3 per cent of the white population in the asylums of Massachusetts consisted of Irish born although they represented only 29.5 per cent of the local population. In New York the corresponding figures were 40.3 per cent and 22.4 per cent. In Connecticut the proportion of insane among the Irish was more than double that of any other nationality. For the United States as a whole Irish patients in 1903 represented twenty nine per cent of all foreign-born white persons in the asylums at a time when they constituted only about sixteen per cent of the corresponding white population[38].

The Australian experience was similar. By the 1890s the statistical evidence showed that there was a higher proportion of insanity there among those of Irish birth than among those of other racial origins. In New South Wales in 1894 the Irish insane constituted one fourth of all the insane in the colony whereas they represented only one fifteenth of the total population. A striking aspect of the rate of insanity among the Irish immigrants to New South Wales was that it was four times higher than that among the Irish who remained in Ireland[39].

Sadly, for some the flight from poverty and famine in the emigrant ships of the period had not been the voyage with the happy ending for which they had hoped. Many of those who became insane were destined to spend their lives in the lunatic asylums of Australia and America. Others 'like hunted animals' chose to return to Ireland[40]. Eventually, where America was concerned, they were given no choice. The authorities there, faced with the mounting burden of insanity, decided to send back to their country of origin those who became insane within three years of arrival[41]. Now, against the flow of hopeful Irish emigrants still crossing the Atlantic came the reverse movement of those broken by the life to which they, too, had once looked forward.

It was, at first, a very small trickle; in 1887 five insane persons were landed at Queenstown, a terminus for transatlantic ships[42]. By December 1893 returned emigrants were 'an appreciable element' of the population of Killarney asylum and it was reported that thirteen per cent of the patients in Mullingar asylum had returned from abroad, mainly from America. In Derry asylum the governors were protesting about having to provide accommodation for insane persons not natives of the area who had been sent back through the local port to a friendless welcome[43]. In March 1903 there were at least 1,450 returned emigrants detained in Irish asylums, over seven per cent of the total inmates[44].

It was a pattern that continued in the years before the first world war. In 1909 Cork asylum had a 'considerable number' of returned emigrants due largely to its proximity to the port of Queenstown[45]. The broken emigrant had by now become one of the saddest figures in the asylums of the period. There was some public resentment of the policy of the American authorities and occasional protests. In July 1909 the committee of Clonmel asylum protested about the enforced return of the insane; one of its members complained that they had been 'set mad in America by overwork'. About the same time the *Tuam Herald* indignantly criticised the practice and, referring to the circumstances in which a local man had been sent back to the area, said 'we do not believe that a Chinaman or a Jap would be worse treated . . .'[46]. But at a time when there was not, in any event, a great deal of public interest in the care of the insane these were isolated cries of protest.

Factors contributing to immigrant insanity

For a while one of the most frequent explanations for the exceptionally large numbers of insane among Irish immigrants was that the unsettled, the thriftless and the unstable tended to emigrate in greater numbers than those who were strong and sound of mind. But as the admissions to lunatic asylums in Ireland itself increased, the contradictory argument was put forward as one of the factors to explain that trend viz, that the strong emigrated and the vulnerable remained behind[47]. More recent studies show that the stress of settling into a foreign culture can affect the well-being of migrants in general. For instance, Norwegian settlers in the USA in 1932 were found to be more susceptible to schizophrenia than either their native or adoptive population. It was shown in 1967 that English migrants in the French-speaking province of Quebec had higher rates of mental illness than those who settled in the English speaking provinces[48]. But the toll of insanity among nineteenth century Irish immigrants was so remarkably high compared with that of immigrants of other racial origins that it demands further explanation. The answer almost certainly lies in a variety of social factors uniquely affecting the Irish emigrant of the famine and post-famine years.

On the face of it, the Irish emigrants of the period started off with certain advantages. They spoke English. They were, generally speaking, literate: in 1851 six out of every ten persons in Ireland over twelve years and under forty could read and write[49]. The great majority were of rural origin adopting new countries where vast areas of agricultural land were available for development.

But as the American experience, in particular, shows the problems of the Irish immigrants arose largely from their decision to reject their agricultural background and to seek, as they saw it, a better life in the city. They had left Ireland with that intention. For generations they had depended on the land of Ireland for sustenance but, ultimately, it had betrayed them. While the likelihood of further cataclysmic famines was remote, life on the small holdings of Ireland could, in any event, offer only continuing hardship and little prospect of social or economic advancement. Even if they were prepared to contemplate a rural life in America their very basic manual farming skills left them ill-suited for the requirements of the large American farm[50]. Nevertheless, if they had chosen to work in agriculture, there was no reason why, in time, most of them would not have acquired the methods to ensure their economic mobility. But young women, in particular, were attracted by the prospects that emigration offered of a better quality of life in the American cities. The life-style of the rural female in nineteenth century Ireland was harsh and subordinate at a time when women were gaining in social status in America and Britain[51].

The extent to which Irish immigrants into the United States between 1875 and 1926 set the city as their goal is illustrated by American immigration statistics. Despite their predominantly rural origins only a small fraction presented themselves as farmers or farm labourers, the majority claiming non-existent skills more likely to be acceptable to urban employers. By comparison, almost all Swedish and German farming emigrants of the period appear to have settled willingly on the land[52].

Between 1845 and 1855 alone close to one million Irish, who had never previously moved further than a few miles from their own parish, arrived in New York. They were mostly poor and penniless without sufficient means to leave the immediate area where they had disembarked. They

crowded into the slums of New York and other east coast
cities; and because they urgently needed employment they
took the unskilled and the risky jobs[53]. Their huge numbers
meant that the labour market became highly unfavourable
for the labourer. A worker without skills could be quickly
replaced by another willing to accept lower wages and inferior
working conditions. The Irish were prepared to work for as
little as 75 cents a day. Even then, many of them were frequently unemployed. Unskilled and resourceless, living in the
most oppressive conditions, many of the earlier arrivals
never achieved either occupational or property mobility and
remained firmly at the bottom of the social ladder[54].

It is not surprising that the plight of the Irish immigrant
was soon reflected in various ways in the social statistics of
the period. Until the end of the century details of hospitalised
immigrants show a disproportionately high figure for those
of Irish origin. As already shown their rate of admission to
lunatic asylums was especially high; it was particularly so
where young women were concerned. The Irish also crowded
the pauper houses. From 1849 to 1891 the proportion of
native Irish in the New York City Almshouse was as high as
sixty per cent and dropped below that figure only twice
during the period. They acquired a name for being drunk,
rowdy and delinquent. The Paddy wagons appeared and took
them to swell the populations of the jails[55].

If the nineteenth century Irish immigrants acquired a
name for being madder, drunker and less respectful of the
law than those of other racial origin these were misfortunes
forced on them by the dire circumstances of their lives. They
had come from a life of hardship to one of far greater deprivation; many of them became casualties. There was no
evidence of any inherent weakness in their character;
but it was clear that their shortcomings were aggravated and exaggerated by Anglo-American prejudices against
the Catholic Irish in general. Nineteenth century racial
thinking in Britain about the troublesome inhabitants of the
adjoining island saw them as a flawed, intellectually deficient
race. Even before the mid-Victorian period 'Paddy' and

'Biddy', frequently represented as resembling apes, were well-established troglodyte images in the British mind[56]. Reflecting this view Charles Kingsley wrote during a visit to Sligo in the 1860s:

> I am haunted by the human chimpanzees I saw along the hundred miles of horrible country . . . to see white chimpanzees is dreadful; if they were black one would not feel it so much . . .[57]

The nineteenth century immigrant found that this unflattering image had already preceded him whether it was in Britain, in its colonies, or in America where there was already a large British influence. Public belief in the deficiencies of the Irish was often openly expressed. The Chicago *Post* commented caustically during 1898 'scratch a convict or a pauper and the chances are that you tickle the skin of an Irish Catholic'[58].

The newly arrived Irish emigrants found themselves, therefore, in a hostile environment. They were expected to show certain deficiencies of character and when instances arose they were seen as inevitable and ineradicable. The Irish misfortunes, particularly the high toll of insanity, must be considered against this unsympathetic background. When their oppressive style of life gave rise to mental breakdown, as it undoubtedly did, there was no sympathy or support for the victims. Late nineteenth century public charity in America was penurious in the extreme. In the 1850s new laws forbade public assistance to immigrant paupers except in grim, deterring institutions[59]. Furthermore those, like the Irish, who came from the lowest social strata, could expect little support from their own. Thus, when they entered the asylums, it is probable that they tended to stay there a long time because there was no one outside to help them find their feet again. This would have aggravated the high numbers of Irish immigrants in the asylums of the period relative to those of other race. Nevertheless, it is evident that under extremely stressful conditions the Irish were more vulnerable than other cultures but the statistics can not be seen as confirmation of the prejudiced popular view that they were inherently subject to a strong streak of insanity. Nor has any evidence of that nature been produced in regard to the subsequent generations of Irish-Americans who sprung from the immigrants of these harsh years.

Moral Treatment
– A Pleasant Illusion

The initial development of the lunatic asylum system was encouraged and stimulated by the view that, given the proper setting, moral treatment offered the prospect of cure for many forms of insanity. Some reformers continued to express their supreme confidence in it even when doubts about it must have already been current. Lord Shaftesbury, speaking in the House of Lords in 1852, claimed that, as a system of care, it was 'the great and blessed glory of modern science, which, by the blessing of God had achieved miracles'[1]. It was a grossly exaggerated view. But the miracles to which Shaftesbury referred may have been the disappearance of the depravities and squalors of the earlier places of detention. For while moral treatment was clearly falling short of expectations in the therapeutic sense its basic humanity had, at least, ensured a departure from the harsh methods of the past.

The broad guidelines for the care of inmates were set out in the asylum rules. On admission they were to be 'carefully bathed, cleansed and clad in the dress of the institution'. Subsequently their treatment was to be carried out 'with all the gentleness compatible with their situation'; restraint, when unavoidable, was to be moderate in extent and duration and to be consistent with the 'safety and advantage' of the patients. In no case were they to receive fewer than three meals daily and every effort was to be made to keep them amused and employed[2]. These directives sum up the concept

128

of moral treatment as it was to be put into practice. Its general direction was initially the joint responsibility of the visiting physician and the lay manager, later becoming exclusively a matter for the resident medical superintendent. It represented, in theory at least, the basic manner in which the insane patient was treated in the nineteenth century public asylum. To that broad regimen of care the physician might add such specific treatments as he believed to be beneficial.

In his presidential address to British and Irish doctors at the annual meeting of the Medico-Psychological Association in London in August, 1881, Dr Daniel Hack Tuke reviewed the progress of the treatment of the insane over the previous forty years[3]. It was a frank appraisal that admitted that no really effective therapeutic method had been identified. Remedies rooted in two-thousand-year-old medical concepts such as copious blood-lettings and drastic purgatives had been tried. The use of shower-baths and frequent doses of tartarised antimony and mercury had also been in vogue for a period. Subsequently other measures including injections of morphia and the use of bromides, chloral hydrate, cannabis indica, digitalis and ergot had their advocates. 'Every remedy' said Dr Tuke, 'leaves a certain residuum of usefulness behind it, though failing to fulfil all the hopes raised . . .'.

And what of moral treatment? By now the claims that it was in itself an effective therapeutic agent had become muted. Dr Tuke made no effort to deal with the subject other than making the comment that as a method it gave rise to 'the liveliest feelings of satisfaction'. It was little more than the expected gesture of support for a form of care that had acquired a certain sacrosanctity. Few of those involved in the treatment of the insane were yet prepared to acknowledge publicly that this much acclaimed panacea for insanity had been, in fact, little more than a pleasant illusion. The reality was that even if moral treatment with its emphasis on kindness and understanding had a beneficial influence it had become increasingly impossible to practise in the setting of the nineteenth century asylum. The type of care envisaged by Pinel and the earlier reformers required that the patient be treated as an individual, not *en masse* with hundreds of others. It was necessary, too, for the patient and his therapist to develop a close relationship; an impossibility in the setting of the large asylum.

From an early stage the conditions that had developed in the Irish district lunatic asylum had ruled out a regimen based on the original concept of moral care. Even before the patients reached the asylum they had been dealt with in a manner which hardly suggested that they were being taken into a caring environment. As already explained most patients were detained under legislative provisions which designated them dangerous lunatics when, in reality, extremely few of them were in that category. Because they had been committed by a magistrate they were handed over for transmission to the asylum to the custody of the police who frequently manacled and tied them with ropes. So many complaints were received about the bruised condition in which they were received that the chief secretary felt obliged to write to all magistrates in 1875 urging that the police convey them in a humane manner[4]. In 1869 a police escort conducted, as a dangerous lunatic, an idiotic child of ten years, still in petticoats, diminutive even for his age, a distance of more than 120 miles from Berehaven to Cork[5]. A commentator in the *Journal of Mental Science* at this time compared the transport of patients in the United Kingdom with those in Ireland:

If Jane Smith becomes the subject of the disease termed insanity she is quietly taken in a fly to the county asylum accompanied by the relieving officer and a female nurse. If, however, poor Biddy O'Callaghan becomes the subject of the same disease she is given into the custody of two police constables in uniform, with their bayonets hanging from their belts, placed on an outside jaunting car and driven through the streets, it maybe, of a populous town to the district hospital for the insane where she is committed as a 'dangerous lunatic'[6].

It was a narsh introduction to a life that would often be devoid of any great show of comfort or kindness. The rapidly increasing patient populations and the overcrowded conditions have already been described. As the asylums grew in size in order to cope with the demands made on them the local governors became increasingly concerned about the cost. With more reluctant financing policies came diminishing standards of comfort. In 1857 the inspectors reported that generally speaking there was a deficiency of furniture and 'a certain air of discomfort' in the asylums. It was, however, a situation that the inspectors defended as appropriate enough for patients who, in the main, had been 'strangers to the personal comforts of life' and to the 'decencies of civilisation . . . huddled together in these miserable abodes which present themselves in quick succession along our public thoroughfares, on the edge of bogs and the side of mountains . . .'[7].

Not everyone shared the inspectors' complacency and believed that the asylum standards were good enough for the peasant Irish. In 1858 the report of the royal commission established on the initiative of Edward Horsman, the chief secretary, provided a graphic and more concerned account of Irish asylum conditions[8]. The commissioners included two members associated with the English lunacy administration and thus in a position to comment with authority. In Limerick and Omagh they found some of the patients 'ill-clad and in a most filthy condition'. In Maryborough the patients had their food tossed out in front of them 'as if they were cattle or pigs'. There was a general disregard in most of the asylums of the rules about restraints which required that only the manager could authorise them. In Armagh a male patient strapped on his back to a bed was, when liberated, 'very feeble, unable to stand, with pulse scarcely perceptible and feet dark and cold'. A foreign visitor to that asylum about the same time, Dr Workman, superintendent of a Toronto asylum, was similarly shocked by what he saw there. He wrote 'this, I trust, is not only the worst in Ireland but in all the world . .[9]

In general the commissioners found inadequate heating arrangements, bad sewerage and a lack of activity and amusement. Although recreation halls had been included in the newer asylums they were rarely used or had been given over to some other purpose. Little had been done to mitigate the bare and cheerless character of much of the living accommodation:

> In corridor or day-room the lunatic sees nothing but the one undiversified white wall, giving to these hospitals intended for the restoration of the alienated mind, an air of bleakness and desolation more calculated to fix than to remove the awful disease under which it labours.

Those criticisms were accompanied by recommendations for a lesser role for the visiting physician and reduced powers for the inspectors. Nugent was stung by the report which he rightly interpreted as casting aspersions on the manner in which he and his colleague had been overseeing the asylums. He circulated widely a printed attack on its findings claiming that the commissioners had deliberately set out to find fault and had not given credit where it was due. And in an unprecedented attack by a government official on a royal commission he alleged that Sir Thomas Reddington, its chairman, had never looked inside the walls of the asylum of which he himself had been a governor until he had visited it on behalf of the commission. Nugent obviously felt that his attack could safely be carried out without putting into question his normal reverence for those in authority. Reddington, a County Galway landlord and former under-secretary of state for Ireland, was a failed politician of little influence. As indicated earlier Dominic Corrigan, the medical member of the commission, had disagreed with some of its findings and Nugent would have preferred to align himself with this distinguished member of his own profession and influential president of the Royal College of Physicians of Ireland. Furthermore, opposition, for any reason, to a report devised to a large extent by Englishmen and likely, if taken seriously, to lead to further Irish taxation could be expected to command a wide spectrum of sympathy. This it achieved. Nugent secured, among others, the support of *The Nation*, organ of nationalist opinion and normally unsympathetic to officials of the Crown.

There was a general raising of hackles; political insults were distributed; but the issue of the conditions of asylum patients remained in the background. Nugent's campaign against the report ensured that it would make little difference to the settled order of things[10].

Staff shortcomings

While the overcrowded conditions and the paucity of funds were the main causes of the poor conditions in the asylums they were aggravated by the personal shortcomings of the staff. In addition to the resident medical superintendent and the visiting physician the only person with professional skills in most asylums for the greater part of the nineteenth century was the apothecary. He was normally non-resident but attended daily to compound medical prescriptions. Later the asylum rules permitted the post of a medical assistant to the superintendent but at the end of 1873 only four asylums had such posts[11]. By the 1890s however the rules insisted on at least one assistant medical officer in every asylum[12]. But even with this post it is obvious that the medical skills available to the asylums had to be spread very thinly over the hundreds of inmates and that care when given depended mainly on the attendant staff.

Professional nurses of any category were unknown prior to the 1860s. Nursing had for long been a disreputable profession carried on by women who often combined it with prostitution. When Florence Nightingale's care of the wounded on the battlefields of the Crimea eventually led to the foundation of a school of training for nurses at St Thomas's Hospital, London, and to the emergence of well-trained, disciplined nurses of good character it represented a notable advance in the development of hospital care. Yet, with the exception of the voluntary general hospitals, nursing in Ireland during the subsequent fifty years remained largely in the hands of untrained personnel, some of doubtful character. Outside the city areas most of the physically sick were cared for in workhouse infirmaries where many of the 'nurses' were unmarried mothers, relatively long-term inmates of the workhouses to which they had been driven by a disapproving society.

The absence of a nursing profession and of respect for nursing was only one of the factors influencing the nature of the subordinate staff recruited for the asylums. There was, to begin with, no clear acceptance that the nature of their duties was in the realm of nursing; and as the concept of moral care receded into a regimen of confinement it seemed more appropriate to think of them as requiring the characteristics of jailers rather than nurses. Since nursing was, in any event, seen as an entirely female activity this was particularly true of the male attendants who were recruited for their physical strength and capacity to restrain difficult male patients rather than for any more tender traits of character.

Initially the male attendants were called 'keepers' and the female attendants, despite their absence of training, were known as 'nurses'. The keepers were responsible for the personal care of the male lunatics; the nurses looked after the female inmates but were also required to clean the male wards, thus being placed in a position of inferiority to the male staff[13]. This was reflected in their pay. In Ballinasloe in 1846 the keepers received twelve guineas annually while the nurses were paid half that amount[14]. The female staff were not allowed to give any personal care to the male patients. It was an arrangement reflecting Victorian sexual attitudes. They are exemplified by a pamphlet proposing guidelines for the operation of asylums drawn up in 1848 by Eyre Kenny, superintendent of a temporary asylum established at Islandbridge, Dublin, to relieve the former Dublin House of Industry of its lunatics. He wrote:

I have long been of the opinion that no female servants should be involved in male divisions . . . the incitement to licentious thoughts and feelings which the presence of females serves to arouse should be guarded against by some such regulation[15].

By the end of the century the 'keepers' and 'nurses' had disappeared. All staff were known as attendants and if Kenny were still alive he must have been happy in the knowledge that by then female staff could not enter a male ward without special permission[16]. It also became settled practice to keep male and female patients apart at all times although during the 1860s they were allowed to dine together 'with great success' in Kilkenny and Sligo asylums[17]. But in most asylums sexual segregation continued to be firmly insisted upon until very recent times.

While employment of any sort was scarce in nineteenth century Ireland work in the asylums was scorned because of the arduous duties and the conditions generally. The parliamentary committee of 1843 reported difficulties in getting 'intelligent and well-informed' attendants, especially females. A new resident physician in Clonmel Asylum had, after his appointment, to remove most of the attendants for 'drunkenness, cruelty and neglect of patients and a total disregard of order and discipline'. There was similar evidence from other asylums[18]. Information furnished to the commissioners of enquiry who reported in 1858 was no different. There were frequent cases of drunkenness in the Richmond asylum. John Mollan, its visiting physician, claimed that most of the attendants were unsuitable for the care of lunatics and were incapable of communicating information to him about the condition of patients. Instances of violence were reported by the asylum's chaplain[19].

The main obstacle in the way of improving the quality of the attendants was the determination of governors to keep down the costs of the asylums. As they grew in size and more patients were admitted there was growing reluctance on the part of the governors to add to the burden of the tax payer by improving the conditions of staff. John Blake, an Irish member of parliament, claimed in 1861 that attendants were being selected with a false sense of economy from individuals ill-qualified by intelligence, education or previous occupation. He had frequently seen the posts given to men worn out in other services such as pensioned soldiers and policemen. The same standards were applied to the selection of female staff[20]. All were obliged to work day and night and most of them were required to sleep in the wards with the patients. In the Central Criminal Lunatic Asylum in Dundrum it was reported in 1891 that staff never had a clear day off duty except when on annual leave[21]. In the 1890s the great majority of Irish asylum attendants were working for wages which varied from one third to one half of those of similar staff in British asylums. There was not a standard ratio of staff to patients; it varied from asylum to asylum and in some places in 1891 was as low as one attendant to twenty patients[22]. When they retired they received, at the discretion of the asylum governors, a pension which was often of the order of four pence a day. While some medical superintendants agitated for better conditions for them[23] in general they received little sympathy from the ratepayers or public representatives.

A big deficiency in the staff was the absence of any training. Irish asylums were not unique in that respect. Prior to 1879 no asylum in the world possessed a systematic programme of training for its staff. In that year Dr Cowles of the McLean Asylum, Massachusetts, instituted the first training school for attendants of the insane. During the subsequent decade training programmes were launched in a number of Scottish asylums and in 1885 the Medico-Psychological Association published *The Handbook for Attendants* which, amended from time to time, was to become over the next thirty years the main source of information for Irish asylum staff[24]. In the 1890s Connolly Norman of the Richmond asylum insisted that attendants seeking promotion should pass an examination; but the Richmond was not typical and up to the end of the century there were few trained staff in the asylums[25]. Most of the resident medical superintendents appeared indifferent and to be of the view that a little knowledge would have been a dangerous thing for staff of such low calibre.

Lack of activity

To the drawbacks of poor quality staff and overcrowded conditions was added the day-long inactivity which appeared to have been the routine of many patients, even those who would have benefited by some form of occupation. Returns for the asylums in 1868 showed that on average about half the patients were employed, the men mainly on horticultural or agricultural work and the women on needlework and miscellaneous duties in the asylum[26]. But it was probably an over-statement of the position; following their visits to the asylums the inspectors of lunacy frequently found it necessary to urge in their annual reports that there be greater activity, pointing out that there was 'nothing recuperative in idleness'[27]. In many cases the amount of land attached to the hospitals was, initially, quite small so that as the asylum population grew it became harder to provide enough outdoor work for them. During the 1880s and 1890s, however, the cost-conscious governors found that asylum farms could be profitable and there was a substantial acquisition of additional land. From 992 acres in 1887 the acreage increased to 2,986 in 1899[28]. But even then there were limitations on the numbers suitable for productive work on the farms and the clear impression given by the inspectors' reports was that a great many patients spent a daily life of inactivity. A notable exception during the 1890s was Mullingar asylum where there was an 'open-gate' policy and many patients went out to work for local employers. Clothing was produced within the asylum that compared well with that of 'the best manufacturers'. For amusement there was a band, weekly dances, cricket and hunts within the grounds with a pack of Bassett hounds[29]

Lalor, Norman and the Richmond Asylum

The Richmond asylum was a notable exception to the air of

pessimism and inactivity that settled on most of the district asylums during the latter decades of the nineteenth century. It had not always been so. Unfavourable evidence was given about the asylum by various witnesses who appeared before the royal commission of 1858[30]. Patients were still being punished as they had been in the eighteenth century by being plunged into baths. Little activity was provided. The apothecary, Pakenham Beatty, had bought a fiddle and a chess-board for the patients' amusement at his own expense. When he also purchased some books including *The Last of the Mohicans* and *The Irish Penny Journal* he was reprimanded and reported to the inspector of lunacy for circulating books of 'a controversial nature'.

Some of the problems of the Richmond asylum derived from the fact that, with over 600 patients, it was by far the biggest asylum in the country and that it had remained until 1857 under a lay manager who appears to have been treated in a most servile manner by the board of governors. Following the appointment of Dr Joseph Lalor as first medical superintendent there was a gradual transformation in the institution's regimen which was to advance it to the forefront of Irish and British asylums. Lalor believed that education and work training were essential to the care of the insane; to him they represented moral treatment in its most effective form[31]. Starting with a school mistress already on the staff he set about extending the education service which he combined with industrial employment and gymnastic classes varying the programme according to the category of patient. His efforts required a special commitment; for many years the governors treated him as they had his lay predecessor and refused to allow him to be present at meetings of the board. His place as its principal medical officer was in fact usurped by one of the inspectors of lunacy who attended the meetings[32].

Lalor, who occupied the post until he died in 1886, became one of the best known asylum superintendents in Britain and Ireland; and the Richmond asylum under his influence became widely known for its enlightened methods of treatment. His contemporary, Dr Daniel Hack Tuke, in an account of British and Irish asylum services described Lalor as, 'a credit to Ireland' and wrote that his system of employing and training the patients was more efficient than anything he had seen elsewhere[33].

Lalor was succeeded as superintendent by Dr Connolly Norman, formerly of Monaghan asylum, Norman, another dedicated doctor, adopted Lalor's educational approach with enthusiasm. But he found that the overcrowded conditions of the Richmond, with about 1,500 patients at the end of 1892, militated against effective treatment in any form. He wrote:

> The huddling together of vast crowds of people anywhere is demoralising; the crowd is apt to take its tone from its worst and not from its best elements ... Recovery or even betterment is often thus impeded or lost and the vicious circle goes on without end ...[34]

Norman was the first Irish doctor publicly to campaign against the futility of asylum detention as an effective form of therapy for many cases of insanity. He believed that the environment of asylum society was essentially an unhealthy one which by fostering a lack of human interest in the broader world simply helped to maintain insanity. He suggested in many papers to professional journals and medical conferences that insanity did not necessarily require the discipline of an asylum and that it should be treated as far as possible in a family setting. He had been influenced in particular by a system in operation in Berlin where patients were boarded out or treated in their own homes and could, when necessary, return voluntarily to the asylum without certification or legal formalities[35]. He would have been aware, too, of the benefits claimed for the long-established practice in Gheel in Belgium under which patients received in the local asylum were dispersed among local families and shared their ordinary life with them. A code of law administered by the burgomaster provided for their protection and supervision. The Gheel tradition was said to have had its roots in the healing influence of St Dympna, believed to be of Irish origin, whose tomb was found locally in the thirteenth century[36].

Norman, in putting forward these views, was many years in advance of his time. Irish policy for the insane, as it was in Britain, was by now firmly based on the belief that a custodial setting was the proper place for them. Those in a position of authority and influence were unlikely to be diverted from that view. It was a policy strengthened by indifference, ignorance and the by now well-established stigma attaching to the family of the patient. It is doubtful whether Norman's views received any serious consideration outside the professional conferences at which he postulated them; the governors of the Richmond reacted to his complaints about overcrowded conditions by extending the asylum and building an auxiliary asylum at Portrane[37]. He later persuaded the new management committee of the asylum to send a deputation in 1901 to Ashbourne, the lord chancellor for Ireland, pressing for legislation to allow a system of family care to be implemented. But they 'did not obtain a particularly favourable hearing'[38]. In time, care within the community and voluntary admissions would emerge as the normal treatment of mental illness but that time was still a long way into the future.

The asylum at the end of the century

As the nineteenth century drew to a close the district asylum was firmly ensconced as a rather harsh and forbidding institution surrounded by high walls commanding little public interest or sympathy. Despite the criticisms of various governmental bodies of enquiry about the poor standards of care little effort was made to advance them. In 1862 the average annual cost of caring for a patient was £21.2.8; in 1891 it was £22.16.2[39]. The governors remained parsimonious at all times. Even with the inducement of a grant-in-aid from central funds of four shillings weekly for each patient, the equivalent of almost half the average cost, it was impossible to encourage them to create kinder and less spartan surroundings. Apart from their concern to protect the local rate-payers, they believed, as they always had, that the standards they had set were adequate for patients who were almost entirely pauper in origin. The inspectors reporting in 1892 on the attitude of the governors wrote that while they wished to treat their lunatics something better than ordinary paupers 'they cannot see the necessity for anything more than the plainest buildings and simplest dietary for patients whose domestic condition and surroundings were in many cases previous to their admission to asylums squalid and poor'[40].

It was a stance prompted by the general attitude of the tax-paying better-off classes towards the financing of services for the poor, the sick and the homeless. The gradual demise of *laissez-faire* and the first manifestations of the welfare state had been painful and alarming events for those who had to foot the bill. The discovery that the number of insane persons needing care was vastly in excess of that originally anticipated was but one factor. A far more serious one was the consequences of the introduction of the poor law system in 1838. George Nicholls's estimate that paupers seeking admission to the new workhouses were unlikely ever to exceed 80,000 was quickly overtaken by the catastrophe of the great famine. In July 1849 there were 222,000 persons in the workhouses and their auxiliaries and a further 784,000 on outdoor relief[41]. While the passing of famine conditions led to a rapid diminution in these numbers the experience had been a shattering one for the rate-payers and had served to bring home to them the hazards of accepting public responsibility for social distress in any form. Pauperism remained high throughout the latter half of the nineteenth century; in 1888, for instance, about 400,000 persons passed through the workhouses and a great many others received outdoor relief[42]. The populations of some rural areas lived scarcely above subsistence level even at the best of times. By the end of the century there were no longer Irish reformers of any importance or influence seeking improvements in the public institutions already provided. It would not have been a popular campaign. In any event political fervour and public agitation were by now almost entirely preoccupied with the issues of home rule, agrarian reform and the dissentions arising from the tragedy of Parnell.

As far as the insane were concerned the optimistic expectations aroused by the initial advocates of moral treatment had vanished completely. Even with favourable conditions the harsh reality was found to be that many of the insane were not curable. In 1859 the inspectors were acknowledging that it would be erroneous to believe otherwise; they reported, 'fully two thirds of the primarily affected are likely to continue so, or from relapses to merge into the state of dementedness'[43]. As the asylum populations grew older, death, rather than cure, became the most likely occasion for the ending of confinement. By 1905 there were 1,450 annual deaths in district asylums compared with 1,389 discharges of recovered patients[44]. The cruelties and abuses associated earlier with their incarceration had gone but the end-of-century district asylum fell very far short of the kind and compassionate setting which the early reformers had in mind. Burdett, the contemporary English authority looked critically at the Irish asylums as the Victorian era drew to a close[45]. It was a familiar recital. He found that 'a spirit of economy exists which would not elsewhere be considered consistent with due provision for the insane'. He wrote of the general frugality, the harshness and wanton ugliness of the buildings, the flagged corridors, the primitive heating and ventilation, the 'truly shocking' conditions of the sanitation, the bareness and gauntness, the all-pervading reminders of the prison and the almshouse. He blamed the former inspectors of lunacy and the 'quiescent' boards of governors:

> The real origin of the present state of affairs must be sought in the failure to arouse and educate public opinion on the part of those whose function it was to have been incessant, in season and out of season, in urging on the public the plain duties that are owing to the insane.

Changing times and changing personalities made little difference and the public were to remain unaroused and uneducated for a long time to come.

The Lunacy Laws Evolve

The law in regard to Irish lunacy matters developed in an unsystematic and somewhat careless manner and by 1890 thirty statutes introduced during the previous seventy years were still in operation to the great confusion of all who had to interpret them[1]. Altogether there had been about fifty separate enactments on the subject but some of them had a short life and had been repealed. This profusion of legislation arose mainly from the fact that the government had moved into a newly developing and previously uncharted area of public activity. Because it was uncertain of the financial and social implications of what it was doing a certain amount of legislative trial and error became unavoidable. With the exception of chancery laws for the protection of insane property owners, few of the provisions were prompted by a concern for the rights of the individual. The main motivating force behind much of the legislation was the desire to limit the financial burden of insanity on public funds and to control admissions to over-taxed accommodation. It was, to a lesser extent, related to ridding the gaols of lunatics.

As described earlier the Act of 1821 had provided for the drawing up by the privy council of rules governing the operation of the asylums. The first rules promulgated in 1843 required that admissions be subject to the direction of the governors following application to the manager. The application had to be accompanied by a medical certificate of insanity and by an affidavit from the next-of-kin declaring the poverty of the patient. They also had to enter into a bond undertaking to remove the patient from the asylum when requested. No provision was made for paying patients[2].

The rules were not, however, the only method of admission. The public outcry that followed the killing by a wandering maniac in a Dublin street of a director of the Bank of Ireland named Sneyd resulted in a special statutory provision being made in 1838 for the detention of dangerous lunatics[3]. It empowered the committal to gaol and the subsequent transfer to an asylum, if the accommodation was available, of any person considered to be a dangerous lunatic or dangerous idiot who had been discovered 'under circumstances denoting a derangement of mind and a purpose of committing some crime'. The committal to 'strict custody' for an indefinite period was made on the order of two justices of the peace after they had obtained a medical opinion. Detention could be terminated only be certain specified judicial persons.

Despite the fact that it branded the patient a dangerous person and a potential criminal this latter method of com-mitting a patient to care became a popular one. It had certain attractions for the family of a patient anxious to be rid of him without any further liability. All dangerous lunatics were treated alike and since proof of poverty did not arise a family in a position to pay for care could avoid having to do so. No undertaking had to be given to accept the patient back into the family but, in any event, committal under this procedure could be tantamount to a sentence of a life-time behind walls. Furthermore, once the justices had ordered detention a place had to be found in a prison or asylum thus avoiding the uncertainty of an ordinary application to an asylum where the governors would have only a limited number of places to allocate among the many seeking them. Yet another attraction to 'friends' of patients was that once the judicial order was made the police became responsible for conveying the lunatic to the place of detention whereas, under the ordinary method of admission, transport was a matter for the family and friends.

This legislation became subject to wide abuse and there

was great laxity in its administration by the justices. Docile persons were treated like dangerous maniacs. Lunatics were encouraged by their friends to commit minor acts of violence so as to provide an excuse for their commital. Some poor law unions availed themselves of the new law to have lunatics transferred from workhouses to gaols thus relieving the workhouse of the expense of caring for them[4].

An important defect in the legislation was that it was tantamount to a reversal of the efforts being made to remove insane persons from a prison to an asylum environment which had been the main thrust of government policy over the previous twenty years. The parliamentary committee of 1843 described it as a 'distressing' example of mistaken legislation[5] and Lord Monteagle protested about it in the House of Lords[6]. The government, accepting the criticisms and anxious to reduce the number of lunatic admissions to the gaols, secured the passage of amending legislation in 1843[7]. The new provisions aimed to curb committals by requiring at least one credible witness to present evidence on oath about the degree of derangement and criminal intent of any person for whom commitment was sought.

In the absence of an adequate number of district lunatic asylums it was not yet possible to end all committals to gaols. By 1867, with various new asylums in operation or about to open, the government felt in a position to take that step. An amending Act provided that a dangerous lunatic or idiot found in the circumstances described in the provisions of 1838 could be committed by the justices only to an asylum subject to a certificate from a dispensary doctor as to his dangerous condition. The system of discharging dangerous lunatics was also simplified. They could be discharged on the certificate of the medical superintendent or visiting physician without reference to a higher authority[8].

With only minor changes this new procedure for the admission of so-called dangerous lunatics remained in operation for almost eighty years until it was replaced by the provisions of the Mental Treatment Act 1945. Over the period a substantial number of all asylum patients came to be admitted in this way. The justices of the peace frequently signed the necessary legal forms without any regard as to whether the condition of the patient was such as to place him in the 'dangerous' category or as to whether he was insane at all. In many instances they never saw the patient nor had any personal knowledge of him. The facility with which individuals could be placed behind the locked doors and high walls of the late nineteenth century and early twentieth century asylum was such that many took advantage of the situation to get rid of friends or relatives who were a burden or a nuisance. This practice has been described earlier. There developed a public complaisance with the asylum becoming a depository for all the unwanted in the community which was to continue well into the present century.

If this practice troubled the minds of those in authority it was not usually because of violence being done to the dignity or rights of human beings. More often it was because the laxity of the justices of the peace was giving rise to what the inspectors termed 'uncalled for county expenditure and continuing trouble to the Executive'[9]. By 1875 about fifty per cent of all admissions to district asylums consisted of 'dangerous lunatics'. This had increased to sixty-six per cent at the end of 1887 when the comparable figure for Scotland, where there was a more complex admission procedure, was only 0.4 per cent[10]. During 1881 an attempt was made by Mr E.F. Litton, the member for Tyrone, to put a private member Bill through parliament which would have introduced more enlightened admission procedures and based British and Irish lunacy laws on the same principles. But the government spokesman was discouraging and concerned about its possible cost to public funds. The Bill was withdrawn[11].

In general the plethora of nineteenth century legislative provisions had little impact on the quality of care of asylum patients. The Lunatic Asylums (Ireland) Act 1875[12] represented an important departure from settled practice and authorised the admission of private paying patients to the district asylums. But they remained institutions where the vast majority of the patients paid nothing because they were paupers or because they had been admitted as dangerous lunatics. At the end of 1894 only 411 patients out of a total asylum population of 12,771 were contributing towards the cost of their care[13].

A report in 1891 by a three-man commission established by the lord-lieutenant to look generally at the lunacy services made a number of enlightened recommendations for changes in the admission laws. Among the suggestions were the introduction of voluntary admissions; the detention of patients only on the authority of a magistrate supported by at least two medical certificates which would distinguish between what the doctor had been told by relatives and what he had observed himself; and a tightening up of the law in regard to dangerous patients. A particularly important proposal would end indefinite detention and limit it to a maximum of three years in the first instance. The commissioners were clearly influenced by the lunacy legislation introduced in 1890 and applicable only to Britain which contained a very comprehensive set of provisions aimed at protecting the rights of patients[14]. But the recommendations were ignored; as far as Ireland was concerned fundamental changes in the laws governing the admission of patients were still over fifty years away.

Criminal lunatics

The first recognition that criminal lunacy required special legal recognition came in an Act of 1800, subsequently amended, which gave power to magistrates to imprison insane persons apprehended when committing a crime. It did not apply to Ireland[15]. However, from the early days of the Irish lunatic asylum system the law provided specifically for the 'criminal lunatic', namely an insane person who had committed a crime or had been accused of one. The 'dangerous lunatic' already referred to was not in this class as he had been discovered only 'under circumstances denoting . . . a purpose of committing some crime'.

The lunacy legislation of 1821 provided that any person

charged with an offence should be acquitted if found to have been insane at the time the crime was committed but it enabled him to be kept in custody during the pleasure of the lord-lieutenant. It also provided that any alleged criminals found insane at the time of their indictment could be similarly detained. Since there was, as yet, little asylum accommodation the gaols became the usual place of detention but the Act enabled transfer of the lunatics to an asylum as soon as a place was available[16].

In 1838 there was a broadening of the concept of a criminal lunatic. Legislation of that year enabled the transfer to asylums of a criminal already undergoing imprisonment, or awaiting transportation, if two doctors certified that he was insane. Prisoners found insane while awaiting trial could also be lodged in an asylum[17].

As the criminal lunacy laws evolved there was a view that they provided loopholes which allowed some criminals who knowingly committed a crime to avoid punishment. The issue was brought to a head when, in 1843, Daniel McNaughton murdered Edward Drummond, secretary to the then Prime Minister, Robert Peel, in broad daylight near Downing Street in London. McNaughton was clearly insane, believing himself to be pursued by devils, and was found not guilty when charged with murder. It was, however, an unpopular verdict and the subsequent controversy eventually led to the definition by the House of Lords of what has come to be known as the McNaughton Rules. They have since provided a precedent in Ireland, as in the United Kingdom, for legal judgments in crimes involving insanity. The rules included a statement that, notwithstanding his insanity, the accused was punishable if he knew what he did was contrary to the law. Furthermore, if a plea of insanity were to succeed the accused person had to be shown to have been insane at the time the offence was committed[18].

The fact that some criminals were now being designated insane did not alter the perception of them in the minds of many as primarily wrongdoers requiring imprisonment in a secure setting. Since in theory, if not entirely in practice, the district asylums were being developed as humanitarian institutions for the care and cure of patients there was difficulty in reconciling with that concept the role now allocated to them of providing prison standards of security for some of their patients. Furthermore while the public at large appeared to have no objection to their 'friends' being committed to asylums as 'dangerous' they were not happy about them being associated with 'atrocious criminals'[19]. When the parliamentary committee reviewed Irish lunacy provisions in 1843 it looked specifically at this issue and at a proposal for a special detached and secure unit within the complex of the Richmond asylum. The committee had before it the views of Lord Chancellor Sugden, head of the Irish judiciary. He wrote:

> Solid objections exist to criminal lunatics being received into district asylums which were never intended for prisoners. The advantage of bringing together all the criminal lunatics . . . is obvious. Their security could be easily provided for, and strangers could be prohibited from visiting that department from curiosity[20].

Sugden's views were accepted and the committee recommended the establishment of a special central asylum. This was given effect to legislatively in 1845 and after various locations were considered it was finally decided to build it on a twenty-one acre site in Dundrum, Dublin. It was opened in 1850 with accommodation for eighty males and forty females[21].

It was the first criminal lunatic asylum. There was, as yet, none in Britain or elsewhere; Broadmoor, the famous English institution, was not founded until 1863. When Lord Shaftesbury, the English reformer and a commissioner in lunacy, was agitating for a similar provision for Britain he claimed within two years of its opening that the Dundrum asylum had been a success[22]. It is hard to know on what basis Shaftesbury could have based so firm a judgment of an asylum which was such a short time in existence. While it was certainly a success in removing from the district asylums and gaols some of the most dangerous of their inmates it was yet too soon to assess its performance as a special asylum. In any event the concept of forensic psychiatry, of specialised care for the criminally insane, was still a long way off given that the treatment of the insane in general was yet largely speculative. Judged in terms of administration, of being a well conceived and efficiently operated institution, the Central Criminal Mental Hospital was far from being a success during its first half century as already shown.

The original concept of a separate asylum for the criminally insane was devised by legislators concerned with the implementation of criminal law. The Irish inspectors of lunacy were, initially at least, opposed to the idea. In their view lunatics in conflict with the law could be adequately catered for in district asylums where, separated from ordinary inmates, they could be given whatever additional surveillance was necessary. They considered that there was nothing extraordinary about the numbers for whom this special provision would be necessary. The annual crime statistics indicated that in the country as a whole there was only a small number of cases where the insane were charged with violent crime. Many others declared to be criminal lunatics by the courts had committed only minor offences which would hardly justify their incarceration in a special asylum. A designated criminal lunatic in Waterford Asylum in 1848 had stolen vegetables valued at threepence; this, it might be noted, at the height of the great famine. Another so-called criminal lunatic languished in the local gaol about the same time for 'having in her possession a workhouse cap'[23].

The statute establishing the new asylum, like some other statutes of the period, was either carelessly drafted or reflected a lack of proper advice in its preparation. Its provisions made no differentiation between minor and major offences. Taken literally it could mean that every person found to be an insane criminal should be committed to the Central Criminal Lunatic Asylum.

Apart from any other consideration this would have been impossible because the number of designated criminal lunatics already in district asylums and gaols far exceeded the places in the new institution. Accordingly, when it was ready for occupation the inspectors selected the worst of those already in detention, a procedure later declared legally acceptable by the government's law advisers. For a period the criterion adopted for referral to the Dundrum asylum was that the lunatics should have been charged with offences involving a punishment of death, transportation or lengthy imprisonment. Later only those who were clearly homicidal or were regarded as dangerous were admitted[24]. Even on that restricted basis the asylum filled rapidly. Because of the nature of the inmates, the discharge rate tended to be low; further accommodation had to be added in 1864, 1884 and 1887 bringing the total places up to 163[25].

The laws affecting criminal lunatics were subsequently amended on a number of occasions. A number of Acts between 1875 and 1884 facilitated the movement of prisoners between asylums and gaols and provided for a special verdict where the accused person was found guilty but insane at the time of the offence[26]. Various early twentieth century enactments touching on criminal lunacy did not make any fundamental changes in the law[27]. By the time the independent Irish administration took over, a substantial body of law had been built up in this specific area. The powers given to the lord-lieutenant in the various British statutes in so far as they referred to the trial and custody of mentally ill offenders were, following independence, transferred to the Minister for Justice[28]. In 1960 the Criminal Justice Act redefined 'criminal lunatic' and introduced new provisions relating to the conditional discharge and transfer of such patients[29].

Chancery lunatics
The earliest statute laws touching on lunacy related to insane persons who possessed property. These laws were rooted in the assertion of England's medieval monarchs that all the land of the realm belonged to the crown. Under the feudal system occupiers of land were granted their estates in return for certain services and for being loyal retainers. If they became incapable of performing these services through idiocy or

lunacy, or demonstrated their disloyalty or untrustworthiness by acts of treason or serious crime, the lands reverted to the crown. A similar practice developed in regard to estates inherited by children during their minority. Were it not for the tempering influence of religious chancellors the early Norman monarchs would have been happy to recover the lands and redistribute them at their will without any regard for the rights or wishes of the former holders. However, the ecclesiastical presence at the royal court ensured the development of practices in keeping with equity and conscience[30].

The original statute law in regard to the property of the mentally unsound was laid down in an Act of Edward I, now lost, but confirmed by Edward II in 1324[31]. It distinguished between idiots and lunatics. The king took custody of the land of an idiot, cared for him out of its income and on his death gave it to the rightful heirs. The king also took over the land of the lunatic, kept it 'without waste and destruction', maintained the lunatic and his household and, if he returned to sanity, gave it back to him. If he died without recovering his sanity the estate was assigned to his heirs and any residual profits 'distributed for his soul'.

The law in regard to wards of court, as they came to be called, continued to evolve through various Acts of parliament which varied somewhat between England, Scotland and Ireland. In Ireland a special commission of part-time members appointed by James I was abolished by him in 1622 when they were found to be allowing 'their friends and dependants. . . to make great gains to themselves in the composition for wardships and other cases'. The king then appointed a court of wards and liveries, patterned on an English provision dating from the reign of Henry VIII, and placed it under the direction of Sir William Parsons, the surveyor-general[32]. It was terminated in 1662 by a hesitant Charles II. He had qualms about ending a measure that gave some influence over the upbringing of young Irish heirs since it was:

very improper to give up that power which the crown
. . . had of breeding them in the Protestant religion by

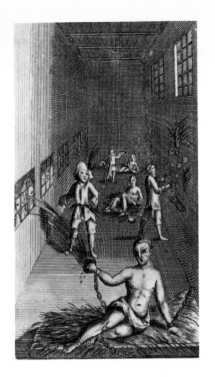
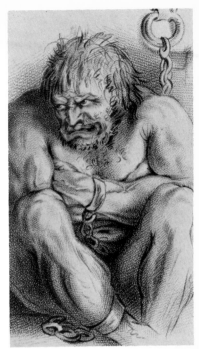
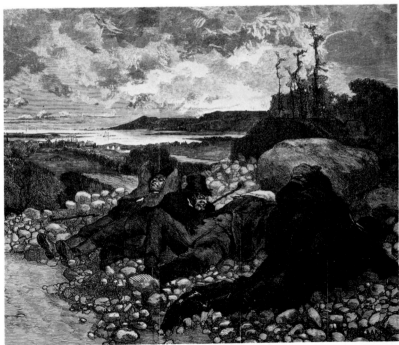

(*Top left*) 18th century lunatic cell from an early edition of Swift's *Tale of A Tub* (*top right*) Madness, from Charles Bell's *Essays on the Anatomy of the Expression in Painting,* 1806 (*bottom*) 19th century continental image of drunken Irish peasants.

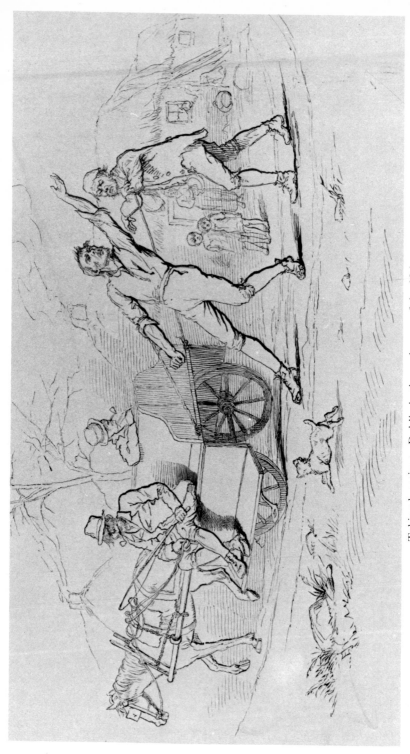

Taking lunatics to Dublin in the early part of the 19th century.

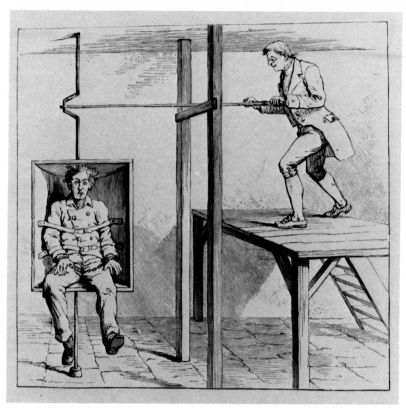

Patients were sometimes suspended in a circulating swing after they had been, 'sufficiently evacuated by purgative medicines' (*p. 59*).

Form of Affidavit, &c. in Cases of Lunatics, whose Friends are desirous of placing them in the Richmond Lunatic Asylum.

AFFIDAVIT.

County of

to wit.

of came before me this day, and made Oath on the Holy Evangelists, that to the best of knowledge and belief has for some time past been in a state of Insanity and Mental Derangement,

is a Pauper, and has no near relative who is able or can be obliged to support in a Private Lunatic Establishment. Deponent further swears that the said been an inmate in any Public or Private Institution for the reception of Lunatics, *

and that Deponent is related to the said in the degree of

Sworn before me at this day of 181

* If the Patient shall have been an inmate of a Lunatic Establishment, here state the place and whether as a Pauper or Boarder.

Physician's or Medical Practitioner's Certificate.

I certify that whom I have visited, is now, and has been, in a state of Insanity for past: I am of opinion that is a fit subject for, and likely to derive benefit from being placed in the Richmond Lunatic Asylum; and said is not subject to Epilepsy.

Given under my Hand, this day of 181

The following Form must be filled up by the Friends of the Lunatic.

Lunatic's Age.	Religion.	Place of Birth.	Place of Abode before Admission.	Occupation, or Trade.	Probable Cause of Derangement.	How long ill before Admission.	Species of Disease.

It is expected that the Lunatic will be sent, provided with a comfortable Suit of Clothes, (and at least) a second Change of every Article. These are to be delivered, marked, to the House-keeper, who will be responsible for their being taken proper care of.

The Forms and Affidavits are to be filled up and transmitted to the Moral Governor, previously to the Lunatic being sent to the Institution; and no Lunatic will be received until it shall be notified to some of his Friends, that there is a vacancy for his reception.

It will be also required that the nearest relative having charge of the Patient, shall sign his consent to the Patient being received into the Asylum.

Form of affidavit and medical certificate required for admission to Richmond Lunatic Asylum, 1815.

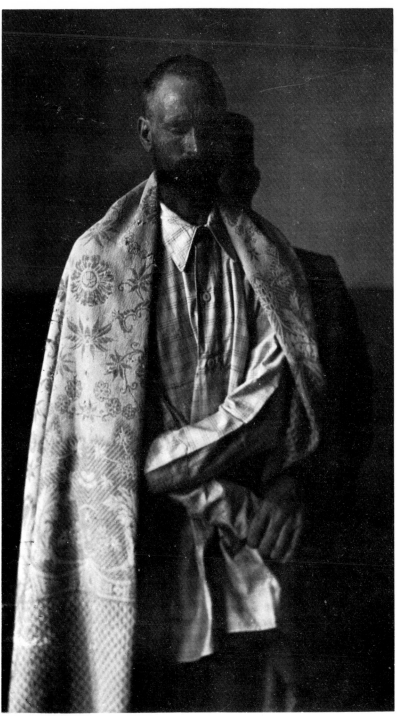

'Moral treatment ... this much acclaimed panacea for insanity had been in fact little more than a pleasant illusion'. (*p. 129*).

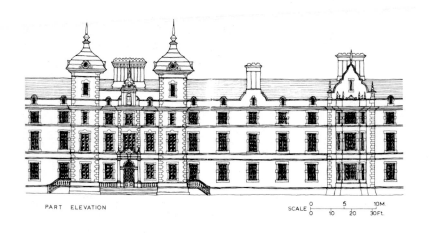

PART ELEVATION

SCALE

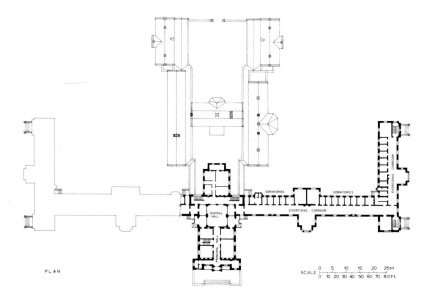

PLAN

Part elevation and plan of St Columba's hospital, Sligo.

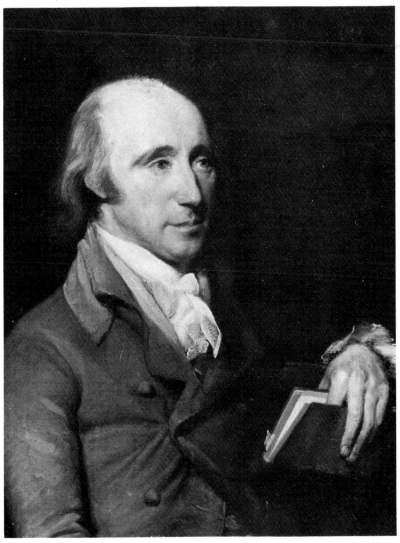

Dr Francis White appointed first Inspector of Lunacy in Ireland in 1846.

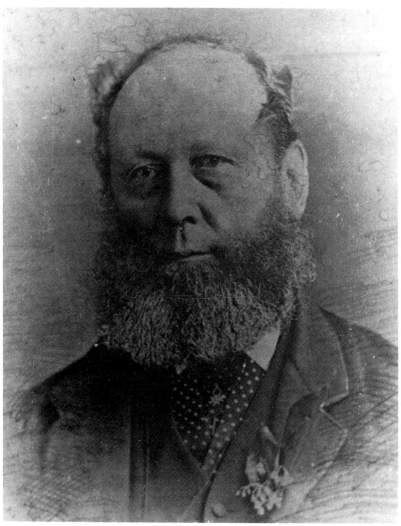

Dr Francis West appointed to manage Omagh District Asylum 1852, one of the first medical managers.

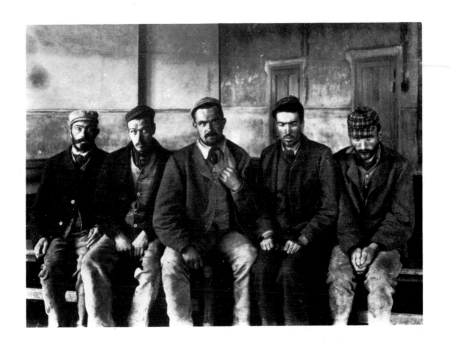

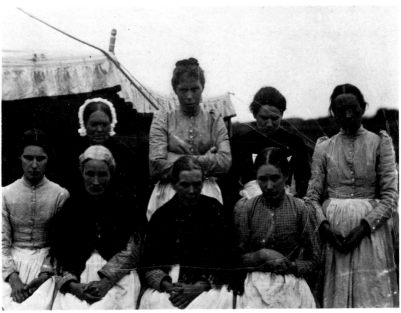

Inmates of a district lunatic asylum, late 19th century.

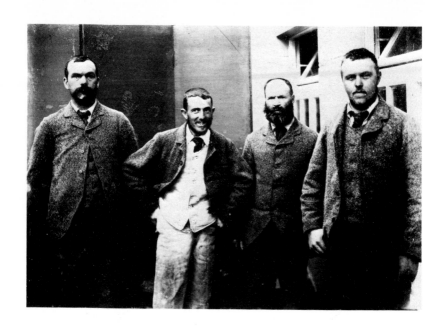

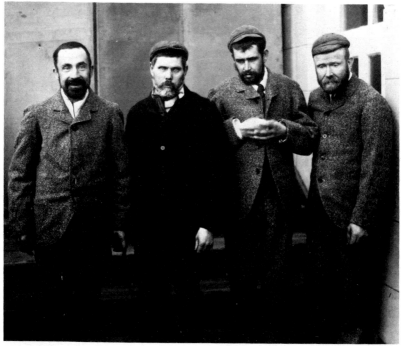

'... overall there was a preponderance of males in the asylums of the Victorian period'. (*p. 111*)

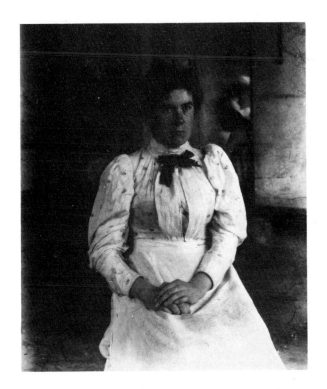

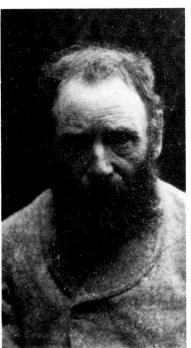

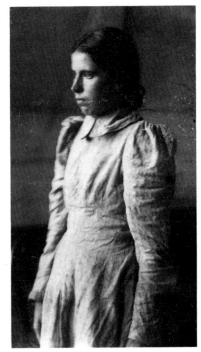

Images of Irish insanity, late 19th century.

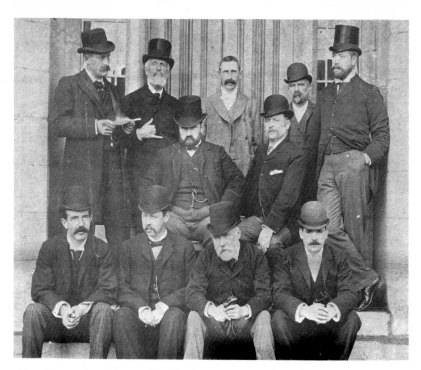

Prominent asylum doctors, 1892 (*back row, left to right*) Drs Norman (Richmond), Patten (Farnham House), Finegan (Mullingar), Pettit (Sligo), Nolan (Downpatrick), (*centre*) O'Neill (Limerick), Woods (Cork), (*front*) Eustace (Hampstead), West (Omagh), Garner (Clonmel), Nash (Richmond).

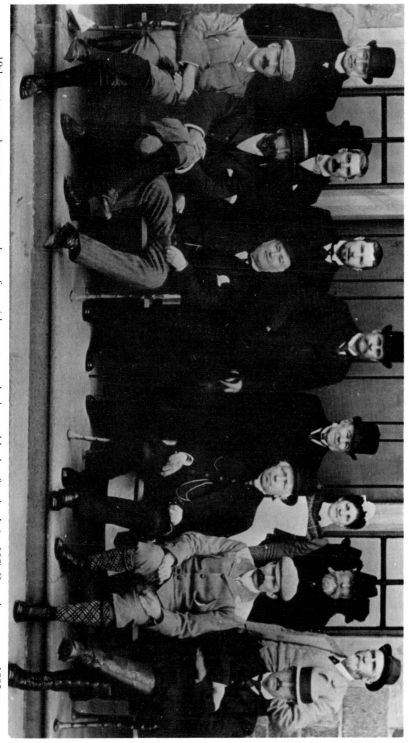

19th century asylum governors were drawn from, 'the gentry and educated body of society'. (*p. 108*) Omagh governors 1895.

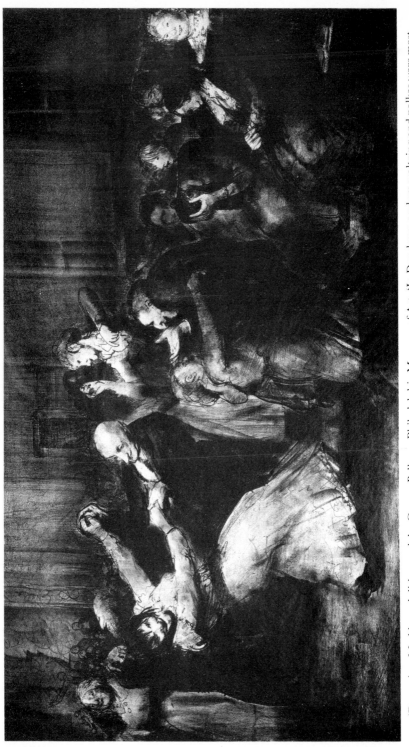

'Dance in a Mad house', lithograph by George Bellows, Philadelphia Museum of Art. 'In Dundrum asylum waltzing and polkas were most favoured' (*p. 102*)

OMAGH DISTRICT ASYLUM.

Time Table for Winter Months,

From __1st__ __November__ 19 __16,__

First Bell
Attendants Rise	-	6-45 a.m.
Patients Rise	-	7- 0 ,,

Breakfast
Attendants' First Table	-	8- 0 a.m.
Attendants' Second Table		8-25 ,,
Serve Patients' Breakfast		8-45 ,,
Patients to Hall	- -	9- 0 ,,

Dinner
Attendants' First Table	- -	1- 0 p.m.
Attendants' Second Table	- -	1-30 ,,
Patients to Hall	- - -	2- 0 ,,

Supper
Serve Patients' Hall	-	5-45 p.m.
Patients to Hall	-	6- 0 ,,
Attendants' First Table	-	6-25 ,,
Attendants' Second Table		6-50 ,,

Patients to Bed

BY ORDER OF THE R.M.S.

Henry Colhoun Storekeeper.

Timetable for winter months, Omagh District Asylum, 1916.

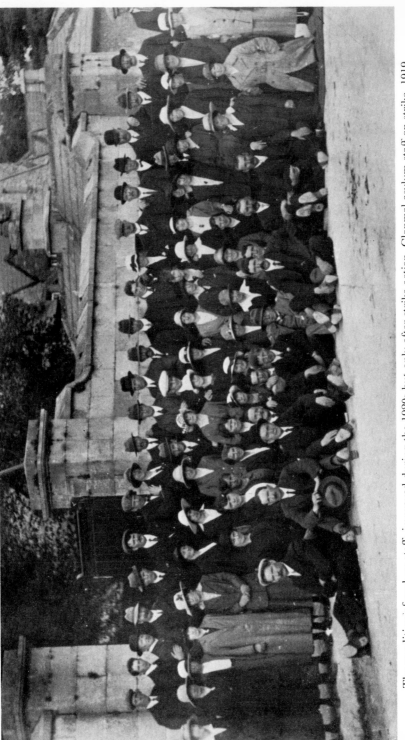

The condition of asylum staffs improved during the 1920s but only after strike action. Clonmel asylum staff on strike, 1919.

means whereof all the great families in the Kingdom might in some time be recovered from the errors of popery[33].

By the middle of the eighteenth century admistrative procedures for dealing with the propertied lunatic had emerged and were firmly established under the direction of the head of the judiciary, the lord chancellor. Heirs and relatives concerned about the mental capacity of an individual to use and protect his property could petition the chancellor to enquire into his condition. If satisfied as to the *prima facie* evidence he issued a writ, *de lunatico inquirendo*, to special commissioners who in turn established a jury to carry out an enquiry into the condition of the lunatic. The jury then decided whether the lunatic's incapacity was such that it was desirable he be designated a chancery lunatic i.e. taken into the wardship of the lord chancellor who would become responsible for the protection and administration of his property[34].

As the nineteenth century district asylums and lunacy laws evolved the lord chancellor's interest and specific responsibilities in this area were recognised. Most of the chancery patients were in private asylums and legislation in 1842 gave him power to revoke a licence issuable under that enactment if he thought it desirable to do so. He was also enabled to direct the inspectors to report to him on any lunatic, chancery or otherwise, irrespective of where he or she was detained even if in the care of a relative. This safeguard for the insane in general was rarely used but is of historic interest because it marks the commencement of statutory safeguards for the detained lunatic which were to be developed in subsequent lunacy and mental treatment laws[35].

During 1843 the then chancellor, Sir Edward Sugden, made a practice of visiting the asylums alone or with the inspector-general. It was the beginning of a period of close personal supervision by successive lords-chancellor of not only the care of chancery patients but of the conditions of all patients in public and private asylums. Most of them followed Sugden's example by visiting the asylums and mingling with the patients. In 1860 an arrangement was begun whereby special medical visitors also inspected the chancery patients and reported direct to the chancellor. By 1892 there were four medical visitors 'of eminence and experience' in the Dublin area and fifty-seven of 'high character' in the provinces. The then registrar-in-lunacy claimed that 'there can be no doubt that lunatics, other than chancery patients, derive enormous advantages from the constant and vigilant attention'[36].

It was probably a reasonable assertion. The close attention given by the late nineteenth century lords-chancellor to the asylums came at a time when no other public figures of power and influence were interested in the subject. Thomas, Lord O'Hagan, during his two periods of chancellorship under Gladstone, 1868-74 and 1880-81 and also in the House of Lords during his interregnum, often showed his concern for the wellbeing of inmates of the district asylums[37]. He was responsible for initiating two Acts of parliament which still form the main basis for Irish law in regard to insane wards of court. An Act of 1871 made obsolete the writ *de lunatico inquirendo* and laid down in considerable detail a new administrative structure and legal procedures for dealing with the estates of insane persons[38]. The post of registrar-in-lunacy was established under the direction of the lord-chancellor and provisions for overseeing the estates of insane wards included the establishment of committees for each estate. In 1880 a further Act had as its object the protection of insane persons possessed of small properties regarded as outside the control of chancery because of the expenses which chancery procedures would involve[39]. This Act afforded protection by vesting jurisdiction in such cases in county court judges.

Lord Ashbourne, who, as Edward Gibson, had served as Irish attorney-general before being promoted lord-chancellor in 1885, also became a frequent visitor to the asylums. Known as 'Tutissimus' among his intimates because of his frequent use of the text, 'Give peace in our time O Lord' he was an energetic and concerned man with a striking appearance which included a crop of silver-white hair[40]. It is easy to visualise the interest his presence must have aroused in the drab overcrowded asylums of the period where a visitor of any significance would have been very rare. He wrote in 1892:

> I have frequent occasion to visit asylums where I converse with all those to whom conversation is possible, and nothing has so much struck me as the immediate recognition by these unfortunate people of the lord-chancellor of whom they have always heard as interested, by virtue of his office, on behalf of the insane. They look upon him as their own judge, their guardian, their protector, to whom they have a right to complain and whose duty it is to listen to their grievances. It is impossible not to be deeply touched with their absolute faith in his power, and many of them hope to believe he will help them, and crowd round him to tell their stories, to make their little complaints, to tell their little grievances, and give utterance to their small and receding hopes[41].

While the unannounced visits to the asylums by lords-chancellor and their network of medical visitors must have had some influence on the standards of the institutions it is probable that they were resented by the central lunacy administration. It is not possible to find any comments in support of the arrangement in the reports of the inspectors or any acknowledgment that they were beneficial. The committee which reviewed the lunacy administration in 1890-91 proposed the establishment of a central lunacy board and queried the need for any special inspection arrangements for chancery patients[42].

Ashbourne resented this view and the fact that the powers proposed for the board aimed 'to silently put aside the whole jurisdiction of the lord chancellor'. The board was not established but, as described elsewhere, much of the responsibility for the administration of the asylum system eventually passed in 1898 to the newly established county councils. The personal interest of lords-chancellor in the affairs of the asylums waned. While the Act of 1871 continued to regulate the affairs of the chancery insane, amending legislation of 1901 made this jurisdiction exercisable by any judge of the Supreme Court to whom it might be entrusted[43]. Following the departure from southern Ireland of the British administration the jurisdiction became exercisable by the chief justice of Ireland and the chief justice of Northern Ireland in accordance with the Government of Ireland Act 1920.

The Recognition of
the Mentally Handicapped

From early times there was an awareness of the distinction between persons now usually referred to as mentally handicapped or retarded persons and those with acquired insanity. Through ignorance or prejudice it was, however, a distinction that was often not made. Persons concerned with the early legal regulation of society or with the care of the sick and the outcast usually recognised the differing origins of mental abnormality. But the common man, and many of the moralists, philosophers and politicians, who from time to time held forth on the subject of madness, often seemed unaware of the difference.

Reference has already been made to the use in the laws of early Irish society of classifications of insanity some of which appear to have related to forms of mental handicap. As also described earlier the first statute law for the protection of the property of the insane dating from the reign of Edward I (1272-1306) distinguished between *idiots*, or natural fools, and *lunatics*. These terms are of Greek and Latin origin; *idiotes* is a Greek word meaning 'a private person' and *luna* is the Latin word for 'moon'. Equivalent terms are to be found in most European languages[1]. In medieval and later times retarded persons were sometimes viewed as *enfants Dieu*, 'children of God'; and allowed to roam the streets of European cities unmolested[2]. As suggested earlier the equivalent early Irish term appears to have been *co rath Dé*, 'with the grace of God' and was probably the origin of the later

157

duine le Dia, person of God. It is reasonable to assume that the suggestion of special divine protection was intended to discriminate between congenitally retarded persons and lunatics during an era when the latter were universally reviled as a manifestation of evil. The distinction was not always respected. Retarded persons were often regarded as figures of fun or amusing freaks of nature. Many were put to death throughout Europe during the witchcraft mania and both Calvin and Luther denounced them as 'filled with Satan'[3].

During the nineteenth century when the mentally retarded began receiving special attention new and vaguely defined classifications were added to the already confused terminology. In Ireland terms such as *harmless lunatics* and *incurables* were often used to describe the congenitally insane but they sometimes included persons with other categories of insanity. *Imbeciles*, *defectives*, *simpletons*, *feeble-minded*, were used at various times to describe categories of retarded persons but definitions varied and it was not until the present century that a settled, generally accepted, terminology emerged.

No matter how they were described the fact that mentally retarded persons represented a distinct form of mental abnormality was recognised by the authorities from the early years of the district lunatic asylums system. The rules issued in 1843 for the operation of the asylums provided that 'idiots, as well as lunatics properly so called, are to be admissable to every asylum, and so also are epileptic persons, where the fits produce imbecility of mind as well as body'[4]. At the same time the Irish constabulary had identified 6,217 members of the national population as 'simpletons or idiots' many of whom were wandering the country 'quite in an unprotected state'[5].

The role of the workhouse
But even then it was evident that the incurable classes were posing problems for the new asylums. The fact that the level of cure of the patients based on the early optimistic expectations of moral treatment was not being achieved; that asylums were packed; and that the discharge rate was low, was blamed mainly on the numbers of idiots who had been

admitted. One of the assistant commissioners working for Whateley's commission during the 1830s had reported following a visit to Ballinasloe asylum, that while the government may have thought it was providing asylums for curable lunatics it was, in fact, 'erecting palaces for the permanent accommodation of slavering and worthless idiots'. It was this situation that influenced George Nicholl's decision, which he later regretted, that provision should be made for them in the newly-developing workhouses. It was a decision influenced solely by the ready availability of the workhouses and the avoidance of further public expenditure. The workhouses could hardly have been regarded as caring centres. They were devised for paupers who in accordance with the philosophy of the poor law were to be constantly reminded of that poverty by an environment that was penal in character. Food and accommodation were spartan. The daily regimen for the inmates was harsh, unpleasant and deliberately 'irksome'. Any suggestion of comfort or pleasure was eliminated. This was illustrated by Nicholl's attitude towards tobacco smoking. He had noted the universal fondness in Ireland for pipe smoking and feared that if permitted in the workhouses it would make tolerable the 'workhouse test', the daily hardships aimed at making the pauper go away. He directed the assistant poor law commissioners who had the duty of inspecting the workhouses 'to look carefully around especially among the old people and every pipe (detected) should be instantly destroyed'[6].

Few, even the most economy-minded, ever considered the decision to associate insane persons, incurable or otherwise, with workhouse paupers to be a proper one. It was not only contrary to the tenets of moral treatment, it was also recreating the worst features of the former houses of industry by intermingling such a wide range of human wretchedness. The parliamentary committee which reviewed the lunacy provisions in 1843 had no doubts about the unsuitability of the workhouses and recommended that the needs of idiots and incurables be met either by extending asylum accommodation or erecting separate provincial centres for them[7]. Boards of governors of the existing asylums were in fairly unanimous agreement with this view. For a while the lord-lieutenant, encouraged by the inspectors-general of prisons, considered the erection in the Dublin area of an asylum for incurable lunatics to serve the province of Leinster[8]. But the concept of separate institutions never made any real progress; the circumstances of the times were against it. The pressure for additional district lunatic asylums to serve parts of the country yet unprovided for had to be met. Furthermore, with the passing of the extreme conditions of the famine, there was spare accommodation in the workhouses and a greater anxiety on the part of the authorities and the ratepayers to avoid additional public expenditure. In addition, White, the inspector, who originally favoured separate institutions, had second thoughts. He came to the conclusion that placing persons in an institution for incurable patients was tantamount to condemning them to 'eternal imprisonment'. It would be more humane to mix them with other patients and to assume that they might recover some time. He would make an exception, however, of the 'most decrepid and imbecile epileptic and idiotic classes' in a large metropolitan area[9]. When the commission of enquiry of 1848 expressed views similar to the earlier parliamentary committee in favour of separate provisions they were ignored[10].

The workhouses, by providing for the majority of the mentally retarded seeking care, now settled into a supporting role for the asylums. It was a role that they were to continue to have over the next century even after their designation as county homes when the poor law system was abolished. At the end of 1862 when district asylum patients totalled 4,506 only 491 of them were described as imbeciles and idiots. At the same time there were 1,268 in these categories among the 2,225 insane residents of the workhouses. Thirty years later there were well over two thousand idiots and imbeciles in the latter institutions[11].

Given the aims of the workhouse regimen the conditions in which the idiots and imbeciles were cared for were always deficient. Sometimes they were housed in 'idiot cells', which were ill-ventilated separate compartments, totally unfurnished, opening out into small yards surrounded by high walls that excluded light and air. Others shared accommodation with the general body of paupers. No special care was given because they had been admitted primarily as paupers and because the workhouse was not organised or staffed to meet the special needs of any of its inmates. When a retarded inmate required to be cleaned or controlled or assisted in some other way the task was often given to a designated pauper who received extras in the way of food or tobacco for his trouble[12]. These often reluctant helpers were themselves persons of serious limitations. Dr George Sigerson, addressing the Irish Statistical and Social Inquiry Society in 1886, described the male assistants as

> . . . men who have been in the lowest rank of unskilled labour, without training, discipline, hope or reward. They have to deal with mentally afflicted paupers — irregular, irresponsible, disorderly and often unclean in their habits . . . it would be impossible to parallel such a condition of things elsewhere[13].

New concepts of care

In the wider world there was throughout the nineteenth century a developing knowledge of the problem and needs of the retarded. Most of the early work was done in France. The basic groundwork on special educational and training techniques was carried out by Jean Itard at the beginning of the century during intensive efforts to habilitate a wild boy found living an animal existence in the forest of Aveyron. Itard worked on the theory that the boy could be brought to normality by placing him in a suitable environment. This belief was based on the mistaken view that intelligence was acquired rather than inherited. While Itard's work was not very fruitful it created an interest in idiocy Jean-Etienne Esquirol was the first to recognise that the basic defect in both idiots and imbeciles was primarily intellectual rather than sensory. There followed a series of educational experiments in France culminating in the publication by Eduor Seguin in 1839 of the first text book on the subject, *The Physiological and*

Moral Instruction of Idiots[14].

With the advent of the first ideas of care came the first special asylums, sometimes called idiot asylums, about the mid-century. They were usually intended for those who could pay. In England small institutions were opened in Bath (1846) and Highgate (1848) and others followed. Similar small-scale developments took place in other European countries and in the United States. Some of those associated with the new movement were remarkably naive and over-optimistic about what could be achieved and created expectations which were not helpful to the movement. Guggenbühl of Switzerland, for instance, held out prospects that the institutional treatment of idiots could lead to normality[15].

The new concepts of care aroused little immediate interest in Ireland. In 1864, however, a small group that included Jonathan Pim, a well-known Quaker philanthropist, and James Wharton, a surgeon in the Meath Hospital, visited various centres for the care and education of idiotic children in England and Scotland. Subsequently one of the party, Cheyne Brady, a governor of the Meath Hospital, published a pamphlet on the subject and a public meeting was convened to consider the establishment of a special institution in Ireland[16]. It does not appear to have led to any action but Pim, in particular, continued to agitate on the subject[17]. In 1866 another group came together at a meeting in the Dublin residence of Lord Charlemont and a committee was set up under his presidency. Its members included Pim, Lord James Butler, John Kells Ingram of Trinity College and George Kidd, a physician in the Coombe Hospital. Kidd subsequently circulated an appeal on behalf of the committee seeking funds to develop a centre which would provide education and treatment for idiotic and imbecile children using methods employed in England[18].

The appeal was not particularly successful largely owing to the fact that the institution was intended exclusively for Protestant children. A sum of £20,000 was required but the subscriptions amounted only to £5,000. Early in 1867 members of the committee went to Belfast where they addressed a specially convened public meeting of prominent Protestant citizens. Pim suggested to the assembly that it would be out of the question having Protestant and Catholic children in the same institution; a reasonable attitude in view of the fact that the ordinary education system was then developing on a denominational basis. He proposed that there should be a single national Protestant institution and he appealed for help from the Ulster counties where, he pointed out, three-fourths of all registered Protestant idiots in the country were located. According to the printed reports the meeting was enthusiastic about the proposals and there were declarations of support[19]. Nevertheless, over a year later, the committee was still far short of the required funds. It was at this stage that Dr Henry Hutchinson Stewart came to its support.

Stewart had been the last governor of the Dublin House of Industry before he ceased to hold office following changes in its administration with the introduction of the poor law system. Under the new arrangements part of the complex of buildings became the workhouse of the North Dublin Union and the hospital areas were placed under separate management. These moves also involved the segregation of almost five hundred insane patients, many of whom were idiots and imbeciles, who up to then shared accommodation with the general body of inmates. Some were transferred to very over-crowded conditions in the Hardwicke Cells associated with one of the units and the remainder were removed to a disused artillery barracks at Islandbridge. The latter centre was closed in 1854 and in 1857 Stewart, who had taken a particular interest in the insane during his governorship, made a contract with the government to care for those remaining in the cells. Under the agreement 101 patients were removed to a private asylum established by him at Lucan Spa House where he undertook to care for them for a payment of £25 annually per patient. Lucan had been a highly fashionable centre noted for its mineral waters but when belief in the beneficial qualities of the waters waned Stewart took over the declining principal hotel and converted it into an asylum[20].

By 1868 Stewart was close to seventy years of age and tiring of operating a large institution but he was in general sympathy with those who saw a need for a special institution for idiot children. He offered to hand over to Charlemont's committee the lease of the asylum at Lucan together with a donation of £4,000. The offer was quickly accepted; the asylum premises together with some adjoining houses purchased from Stewart on favourable terms were taken over towards the end of 1869 and re-organised into two separate institutions. They were the Stewart Institution for Idiots 'based on Protestant principles of the broadest and unsectarian character' and the Stewart Asylum for Lunatic Patients of the Middle Classes in which no religious distinctions were made. The asylum was provided at Stewart's request but the primary aim of the management committee was to make available an education for idiot children. In order to emphasise the educational aspect the children were referred to as 'pupils' not patients. A proportion of the children were admitted free; the others paid the cost of care and those whose families could afford it were provided with separate accommodation and special attendants. The whole institution was placed under the medical direction of Dr Frederick Pim who, in preparation, had spent several weeks studying the methods of some English institutions[21].

The initiation of the project had raised some controversy. The Catholic primate, Cardinal Cullen, saw it as a threat to Catholic children and was not prepared to accept that it was founded solely for the education of Protestants. 'It was founded in an aggressive spirit' he alleged in a letter to the parish priest of Lucan He branded it a proselytising agency and gave instructions that Catholics were not to patronise or encourage it directly or indirectly[22]. The allegations were unjust but must be seen against the background of Cullen's opposition to the widespread campaigns being carried out over the previous decades by Protestant missionary societies in Ireland. Cullen also protested to Lord Spencer, the lord-lieutenant, probably on the basis that many of the more prominent supporters of the institution were government office-holders. Spencer, anxious to avoid any suggestion of government involvement in an activity provocative to Catholic opinion, discussed the issue separately with both Cullen and Charlemont. Charlemont's explanation left him 'quite satisfied'[23]. No changes were made in the rules for operating the institution.

By the middle of 1870 the Lucan premises were overcrowded and the management committee decided to purchase the residence and demesne of the late Lord Donoghmore at Palmerstown. These were acquired for £4,000; the premises were considerably extended, and early in 1879 all the inmates of the Lucan institution were transferred there. The new centre was named the Stewart Institution for Idiotic and Imbecile Children and Middle Class Lunatic Asylum[24]. In time the institution dropped the asylum element, shortened its name to Stewart's Hospital, and became wholly a centre for mentally handicapped children and adults. For almost fifty years it was to be the only special provision of that nature in Ireland.

In the eyes of the public and those in authority lunacy and idiocy continued in practice to be seen in Ireland and elsewhere as largely elements of one problem. Over the following decades there was little progress towards separate provisions. In Britain the Idiots Act, 1886 made specific provision for the admission and supervision of idiots and imbeciles. It was a token recognition that achieved little and was brought about mainly by British reformers such as Sir Charles Trevelyan and Lord Shaftesbury who had been agitating for special recognition of this sort[25].

In Ireland the question of providing separately for idiots received little government attention at this period although official reports continued to draw attention to the need for further provision for them. The workhouse remained the principal depository for them unless they could be abandoned in some other way. The commission of 1879 on the poor law and lunacy systems expressed concern at the freedom with which idiots were permitted to wander abroad 'often teased, often goaded to frenzy by thoughtless children, often the victims of ill-treatment or the perpetrators of offences far worse'. The commissioners had reservations about reports from the inspectors of lunacy that, in general, workhouse idiots and lunatics were receiving reasonable care. Their doubts were understandable in view of the visiting record of the inspectors. Seventy-three of the one hundred and sixty-three workhouses had been left unvisited for three years or more despite the inspectors' duty to visit them regularly[26].

The main obstacle in the way of any improvements or special provisions continued to be the financial one. There was, at this period, growing concern about the cost of lunacy and increased resistance to paying for it. In 1875 the total contribution from public funds, central and local, to the district asylums had been £197,000. Five years later, when the average daily occupancy of the asylums had increased by nine hundred patients, the contribution had actually fallen by several thousand pounds due to reduced grants from local rates[27]. In this climate the commission of 1879 was unlikely to recommend any very radical changes for idiots; on the contrary its proposals deterred asylum improvements which would have contributed to their needs. Its report recommended that all expenditure on new asylum buildings and extensions be suspended and that 'harmless' lunatics, including idiots and imbeciles, be provided for in spare workhouse accommodation. The commissioners also considered that the district asylums should be classified into two categories: lunatic hospitals for those who were curable and lunatic asylums for 'chronically insane requiring special care'. This latter category appeared to include idiots and imbeciles. The commissioners also recommended that dispensary doctors be obliged to supervise the well-being of imbeciles and other insane persons 'at large' and that a medical certificate of neglect or improper care should be sufficient to require action from the lunacy authorities.

In general the recommendations in the report had the familiar fate of being ignored. Shortly before the report was submitted, boards of guardians had been statutorily empowered to transfer insane inmates to any other union that might establish separate provision for them[28]. But the determination of guardians to curb local taxation prevailed, and no measures of this sort were taken. By the 1890s there was a reluctant acceptance by the central authorities that for the time being at least the best that could be done for the insane in the workhouses was to improve their conditions where they were. Efforts were made to ensure that paid, not pauper, staff looked after them; that less use was made of strait-jackets and other restraints; that separate accommodation was provided and idiot cells closed[29].

Transfer to the asylums

There had always been a flow of patients from the workhouses to the asylums owing more to financial considerations than to a desire to secure a better setting for the patients. The pressures now applied to the workhouse guardians to provide an improved level of care for their insane inmates accelerated that movement. In 1891 the number of patients transferred was 381. By 1899 it had risen to 667. Changes in the local authority system gave a further stimulus to the transfers. The Local Government Act, 1898, to which further reference will be made, assigned the financing of the poor law to the new county councils and also transferred to them responsibility for the provision and management of the district asylums[30]. Furthermore, influenced by the earlier commission, the Act enabled the new authorities to establish auxiliary lunatic asylums in selected workhouse premises for the reception of 'chronic lunatics who not being dangerous to themselves or others are certified . . . not to require special care and treatment'. Any auxiliary so established could be regarded as a separate asylum or as a department of an existing asylum. Under these changes the financing of both the workhouses and the asylums became mainly the responsibility of the same authority, the local county council, but central government grants remained more favourable in respect of asylum patients. The rate of transfers accelerated; in 1904 over a thousand inmates were moved from the workhouses to the asylums, a quarter of all admissions[31].

The large-scale transfers of the chronically insane and idiot population of the workhouses led, in one instance only, to a separate provision for them. In Youghal an industrial school was taken over in 1902, extended, adapted and designated an auxiliary asylum. Over two hundred cases were transferred to it from the workhouses of the Cork area[32]. No auxiliaries were opened elsewhere; understandable since the government grant towards them would have been only two shillings weekly per patient, half the rate payable for patients in the main lunatic asylum [33]. In effect what was happening was that the workhouse insane consisting of a large proportion of idiots and imbeciles were now being integrated in the existing asylums and the provisions enabling separate accommodation for them was being ignored. But there was a limit to the number that the overcrowded asylums could accept. Early in 1905 there were still 3,165 lunatics and idiots in the workhouses, some 'excitable and troublesome'[34]. Ten years later reports of the inspectors showed that some of them were still being cared for in a wretched manner. In Ballina workhouse 'the condition of life of the mentally afflicted . . . reveals a state of affairs urgently calling for redress'; in Waterford the evidence of vermin was 'most discreditable to those in charge'; in Belmullet the diet included a thick gruel which the inmates could not eat and which was usually fed to the pigs[35].

The position of idiots and imbeciles elsewhere appeared to be no better than in Ireland. Earlier enthusiasm for new ideas and experimentation had given away to pessimism by the end of the century. Faced with the irreversibility of a congenital condition, attention, when given at all, concentrated on the training of the mildly handicapped to the exclusion of the more severely afflicted. It was facilitated by the formulation at the turn of the twentieth century of Alfred Binet's tests of intelligence which created criteria for the measurement of intellectual capacity. This development enabled the classification of mentally retarded children so as to distinguish between those who were educable and those who were not. It also made possible the identification of mild intellectual retardation in cases where it would not otherwise be discernible[36]. In Britain, but not in Ireland, legislation during 1899 empowered education authorities to arrange special facilities for retarded children unable to benefit from instruction in the ordinary elementary schools[37].

There was sufficient public pressure for better provisions, particularly where children were concerned, to give rise in 1904 to the Royal Commission on the Care and Control of the Feeble-minded. Its report four years later contained the first comprehensive review of the needs of the various categories of persons with congenital mental defects. The commission's remit covered both the United Kingdom and Ireland, and while the basic principles of its recommendations were similar in relation to both areas there were some differences in detail[38].

Four classifications were proposed: idiots, imbeciles, feeble-minded and moral imbeciles (later moral defectives)[39]. Idiots represented the most dependent group while those designated moral imbeciles were described as persons who had a mental defect coupled with 'strong vicious or criminal propensities'.

In its findings on Ireland the commission estimated that there were over 25,000 persons in these classes. It calculated that 7,580 were children, almost all of whom lacked provisions of any sort. One of the barriers in the way of making a special educational service available for them was that the national school system for normal children was still not universally available on a compulsory basis. Furthermore there was not a local educational authority such as in Britain which could carry out the necessary planning and organisation. Irish national schools were usually managed by one person, invariably a clergyman, whose administrative role was a very limited one. Nevertheless ordinary schools occasionally admitted imbecile children to their classes despite the fact that teachers had to cope with very difficult conditions. An investigator on behalf of the commission wrote following a visit to a classroom for infant children in a Belfast school:

> ... on opening the door ... I was compelled to stand back to permit a clearing away of what cannot be

described in less terms than a stench. Greatly to my surprise I found this room literally packed with infants up to six years of age, as tightly as the small benches could admit them, while others were crowded over the floor up to the teacher's feet . . .

There were similar conditions in Dublin schools. The investigator concluded that in regard to the admission of idiots and imbeciles to such schools 'there can be no question whatever as to its futility and worthlessness, not to speak of its undoubted cruelty . . .'[40].

The commission recommended that local authorities be statutorily obliged to make suitable provision for all mentally ill and abnormal persons subject to the direction of a specially constituted central body. The report led to the enactment for the United Kingdom of the Mental Deficiency Act 1913[41] but no action was taken in regard to Ireland. In practice the care of the mentally ill and the mentally handicapped continued to be treated as a single problem over the next fifty years.

From Lunacy to Mental Illness

The position of lunacy in Ireland at the beginning of the twentieth century can be summarised briefly. There were about 21,000 insane persons of all categories in care, either in asylums or workhouses, and the number was continuing to rise. Thousands of others, mainly idiots, resided in their own homes or led a largely vagrant life[1]. Those in the institutions were receiving care rather than treatment. Isolation and safe custody had taken over from moral treatment. Because its clinical dimension appeared to be minimal the management of lunacy was now seen as only peripherally involved with medicine and it operated without any real links with the care of the physically ill. This segregation of mental illness itself helped to strengthen the stigma associated in many minds with the asylum patient. There was, consequently, a ready public acquiescence in the policy of confining the problem of insanity behind high walls both in the literal and the figurative sense and no great inclination on the part of anyone to spend more money on improving the quality of care. There were, however, important scientific, political and administrative developments taking place which, in differing ways, would influence the care of the insane in Ireland.

Beginnings of scientific physchiatry
In Vienna in 1900 Sigmund Freud, who had been studying the origins and treatment of neurotic behaviour, published

171

The Interpretation of Dreams. It represented a major break-through in the understanding of the human mind and was to become one of the taproots of modern psychiatry. Freud had concentrated on the childhood environment of individual patients, particularly their relationships with their parents, and was convinced that neurotic behaviour and personality were determined by these early experiences. In particular he identified various sexual disturbances which he believed to be Oedipal in character. His concepts were elaborated in further publications including *Three Essays on the Theory of Sexuality* (1905). *Mourning and Melancholia* published in 1917 outlined his theories on the genesis of depression. Not all his views were generally acceptable. Some offended current notions of morality and were seen merely as the sexual pre-occupations of a Viennese doctor with a vivid imagination. Other views, notably those concerning depression, brought him into conflict with supporters of ideas advanced earlier by Kraepelin. But even if his ideas were controversial and unacceptable in their entirety they had stimulated a great deal of thought and argument and had opened a new era of psychiatry. Others such as Carl Jung, Otto Rank and Alfred Adler took up his theories and elaborated and modified them. Adler argued the influence of the present rather than the childhood environment on mental disturbance. A whole new body of theory and knowledge developed in regard to the illness of the human mind which was to provide deeper insights into the symptoms and needs of patients. Psycho-analysis emerged as a technique for assessing and treating the individual patient[2]. The new ideas were undoubtedly complex and slow to root; 'I thought he was a little above my head' said one Irish psychiatrist who underwent lectures given by Freud in Vienna during the 1920s[3]. But with Freud and his contemporaries the care of the disturbed mind moved more rapidly away from age-long notions implicit in the term lunacy and towards the recognition of mental illness, a human condition capable of explanation and treatment in enlightened and scientific terms.

Growth of local government

Of more immediate import to the Irish lunacy services were the political and social changes taking place in Ireland during the early decades of the century. If self-determination for the Irish was still some distance in the future the establishment of a new local government system was, at least, a notable advance in the development of universal suffrage and the concept of democracy. The county councils established under the Local Government (Ireland) Act, 1898[4] became responsible for the administration of most local public services including the district asylums. They took over also the powers of grand juries, presentment sessions and poor law guardians in regard to local taxation. The *ex-officio* and nominated elements on local bodies disappeared and membership of the new councils became subject to popular elections. All who possessed a household acquired the right to vote.

The creation of the county councils marked the end of ascendency power in local affairs in Ireland. After 1898 the representation on local bodies of the establishment classes started to diminish while the wage-earning classes began to appear in increasing numbers[5]. The composition of the bodies became a more authentic reflection of Irish society; Protestant dominance, particularly in the control of the asylums, ended in many areas. The Catholic representatives avidly grasped their unaccustomed superiority on the new management committees appointed by the councils. In Sligo in 1908 the county council co-opted six Catholic clergymen, including the local bishop, to the committee of the local asylum. The bishop was made chairman. No Protestants were co-opted[6]. Catholic clergy also became a strong force on other asylum managements. In response the Protestants in the Northern counties strengthened their control of committees whenever it was possible.

It was a period of considerable political excitement. Few people were concerned with social issues. Politicians and general public, north and south, were pre-occupied with the agitation for and against Home Rule. The opportunities presented by the fact that the new local authorities provided not only a public forum for political agitation but had statutory powers that could be used, or misused, to embarrass the government were quickly grasped by the nationalist population. Henry Robinson, vice-president of the Irish Local Government Board during the period, later claimed that 'the first principle of Irish life' was to obstruct the government[7]. This was most effectively achieved by constant resistance by the nationalist controlled local authorities to the Local Government Board. The loyalist areas were not troublesome. Robinson wrote:

> The chief characteristic of northern administration was rigid economy. The members of the local bodies were mainly business people with the Scottish instinct to get value for their money and they kept the rates down and seldom fell foul of the auditor; while the southerners were characterised by a greater openhandedness and more high-spirited contempt for the restrictions of English acts of parliament and had to be closely superintended.

If there was openhandedness it did not extend to the asylums. Now that the native Irish were in charge of the care of their own insane they were no more generous than the ascendency governors who had for so long based their parsimonious management of the asylums on the just rights of property and on the belief that, in any event, institutions for pauper patients should reflect the grimness and discomforts of poverty. Reports of early twentieth century meetings of the new committees of management had a familiar ring. They showed a pre-occupation with financial matters, opposition to wage increases, questioning of expenditure on food and a remarkable lack of concern about the living conditions of the patients themselves.

The attitude of the new committees was, fundamentally, nfluenced by the continued absence of any real public interest in the asylums or their patients. Furthermore, the Local Government Act had set clearly defined limits to support from government funds. As already shown the expenses of the asylums had been met prior to 1898 by a county tax supported by a government grant of four shillings weekly in respect of each patient. Under the new arrangements the asylums became a charge on the county rates with limited support from central funds. The capitation grant, which continued, became payable from the Local Taxation Account, the income of which consisted mainly of local licence duties. It was clearly not intended to be a bottomless purse. The account was limited by its annual income; when demands on it exceeded that income, capitation grants were proportionately reduced[8]. This meant that the ratepayers had to meet the total cost above a certain level of spending; a measure intended, no doubt, to dampen down the 'high spirited contempt' described by Robinson.

The number of insane in care increased steadily between 1900 and 1914 from 21,169 patients to 25,180[9]. Until 1909 the Local Taxation Account was able to meet the total demands but in 1909-10 it was no longer able to do so and the support given to the asylums and the workhouses was abated[10]. This situation had been hastened by the Liberal government's budget of that year when, in order to help pay for the newly-introduced old-age pension, it was found necessary to appropriate some of the funds normally available to support local taxation in Ireland. There were Irish protests and deputations to Dublin Castle but Augustine Birrell, the chief secretary, could only express personal sympathy and pass the responsibility to the chancellor of the exchequer, Lloyd George[11]. Paradoxically, despite the introduction of social provisions that could be said to mark the commencement of the welfare state, the Liberals had simultaneously embarked on a much-vaunted policy of reducing government expenditure[12]. From then until the departure of the British administration from Ireland central government contributions to the asylums remained practically static and any increased expenditure had to be met fully by the local rates[13].

Commissions of 1906-1909

Between 1906 and 1909 three separate commissions of

enquiry reported on services for the insane in Ireland. None was set up specifically to do so; each of the three had a broader remit which brought the Irish asylum system within its ambit. The previous chapter has dealt with the findings of one of them, the Royal Commission on the Care and Control of the Feeble-minded (1908), established principally to make recommendations about the care of idiots and imbeciles. It also urged the ending of the use of the words 'lunatic' and 'asylum'[14] . While the word 'patient' quickly replaced 'lunatic' the 'inspectors of lunacy' continued to operate from the 'Office of Lunatic Asylums' and to report on the 'district asylums' until the ending of British administration in Ireland.

The other two commissions were concerned primarily with the review of the poor law but both examined the lunacy provisions. The Vice-regal Commission on Poor Law Reform in Ireland reported in 1906[15] and was followed three years later by the report of the Royal Commission on the Poor Law and Relief of Distress which examined the position in the United Kingdom and took another look at Ireland[16]. Their findings did nothing to improve the institutional or legal provisions for the insane in Ireland; on the contrary the general thrust of their views may be said to have introduced and justified a period of stagnation which was to continue until after the second world war.

The vice-regal commission had been specifically requested to examine the position of the workhouse insane and to advise whether a system of auxiliary asylums might be provided for them. The volume of evidence favouring their removal from the workhouse was overwhelming; but the motivation of the witnesses was financial rather than humanitarian. The asylum doctors were, however, against the idea of auxiliaries fearing, with good reason, that they would be used to provide a cheap and inferior level of care[17]. Some of them, like Connolly Norman, appeared before the commission to urge that patients would thrive better in the surroundings of family care rather than in overcrowded institutions. But there was hostility from other witnesses to sending them home or boarding them out. 'A new terror will be added to life'

176

declared one witness. Other unsympathetic notes were struck. A justice of the peace from County Wicklow would reduce the level of lunacy by emasculating all male lunatics because of the heredity factor[18].

The commissioners recommended that all insane persons in the workhouses be transferred to either district or auxiliary asylums[19]. No recommendations were made about the possible advantages of family care or about any other innovations which would get away from the prevailing policy of isolation and confinement. The report in general left no doubt about the commissioners' lack of sympathy for any substantial effort to improve asylum conditions. It would, they declared, 'be unnecessary and wasteful' to incur heavy expenditure on additional buildings. Disused workhouses should be used. While they expressed admiration for the efforts of the inspectors of lunacy to arouse sympathy for the insane they believed that the sane sick had more urgent claims on 'the practical sympathy of the ratepayers'. They pointed out that the sick poor were in far inferior conditions in the workhouse infirmaries where they had 'the roughest of beds in unplastered and unceiled rooms and were attended upon by degraded unpaid inmates as nurses'.

There was no doubt about the wretchedness of the workhouse wards then providing the only hospital care available to many sick people in rural Ireland. As already shown the philosophy of the workhouse system as a whole required the creation of an environment which the paupers, sick or otherwise, would find repellant. The fact that the commissioners were able by comparison to see in the grim over-crowded asylums evidence of superior conditions merely emphasised the abysmal quality of the workhouse hospital and the extent to which it was permeated by the degrading principles of the poor law. If a choice had to be made it would have been hard to quarrel with preference being given to the sick poor rather than the insane poor.

One of the most effective and influential witnesses coming before the vice-regal commission had been Dr Kelly, Catholic Bishop of Ross, member of the committee of management of

Cork District Lunatic Asylum[20]. His personal views about public spending on the asylums and workhouses could only have endeared him to the government. He was opposed to the repeal of the 'quarter acre clause', one of the most resented features of the Irish poor law which debarred a person with over that amount of land from getting relief unless he sacrificed his miserable plot. Kelly believed that the existence of the clause was an 'incentive to self-reliance' and that it kept large numbers of the population 'on the right side of the border line which separates poverty from actual pauperism'. His attitude towards public expenditure on social services reflected that of the Catholic hierarchy in general who were unenthusiastic about welfare spending at a time when their first priority was the development of education[21]. Kelly was an advocate of auxiliary asylums which he felt could be run more cheaply than district asylums by avoiding what he regarded as the more expensive traditions of the latter. He saw no need for doctors in the auxiliaries; they could be operated adequately and economically by nuns who then received little payment for their services. He had been the main driving force behind the establishment of Youghal Auxiliary Asylum to which reference has already been made. *The Journal of Medical Science*, mouthpiece of the asylum doctors, commented in 1907 that the staff in that institution was insufficient to provide proper care for the patients who were frequently kept indoors all day; and it protested about the 'retrograde character' of the principles on which the institution was based[22].

The Royal Commission on the Poor Law and Relief of Distress which reported in 1909 had been established four years previously by the Conservative prime minister, A.J. Balfour, just before he vacated office for Asquith's Liberal government. The commission came at a time of considerable discussion about poor law reform in the United Kingdom and its membership included a number of active social reformers of the period, notably Beatrice Webb and Octavia Hill. The Irish dimension in the membership was a small one: Sir Henry Robinson and Bishop Kelly.

The main recommendations of the commission are not relevant to this account; they proposed in effect the abolition of the whole structure of the Irish poor law machinery, a change which came only after the departure of the British administration. The report referred only briefly to the subject of the Irish asylums. It pointed out that the vice-regal commission had already dealt fully with them and had made recommendations; it added succinctly 'with these recommendations we concur'[23].

The Irish findings of the report had been almost entirely influenced by the two Irish members of the commission. Its English members had found it difficult to understand the views and mentality of some of the witnesses who had travelled from Ireland to give evidence when the commission was sitting in Westminster. The choice of witnesses, according to Robinson, had been determined by their willingness to undertake a long, but free, journey to London rather than their knowledge of the poor law. Some rambled incoherently in their evidence[24]. The chairman had difficulty pinning down one witness, a horse-dealer; Robinson describes him giving evidence:

'Well then, I'll drop that and I'll come to another subject. Smokeless powdher. Ay, smokeless powdher. Now the great pint about this is . . .' Here the chairman interposed 'Yes, I quite understand it is, as you say, in itself a most interesting thing, but I'm afraid I must really rule it as outside the scope of our reference. I'm afraid we cannot connect it with poor law reform'. 'I'm coming to that' said the witness, with a wave of his hand; but he had evidently forgotten the connection for after studying his notes carefully he burst out with: 'Oh ay, poor law — now this is very important; illegitimate childher', and then glancing around the table and lowering his voice decorously, he continued, 'now with all respect to the ladies present, them illegitimate childher is a very great mishtake'.

Robinson's portrayal of the witness as a comic Somerville

and Ross type character is clearly an exaggeration. But the commission obviously had problems with its Irish witnesses and decided to visit Ireland to see whether it would help clarify the Irish aspects of its remit on the spot. Dividing into three groups they 'made a hurried scamper' around the country, held one meeting in the Custom House and then left the drafting of the Irish part of the report to Bishop Kelly and Robinson. The commission as a whole later approved the draft with little amendment[25]. It concurred with the earlier views on the asylums of the vice-regal commission, and thereby bestowed its blessing on the continuation of a policy which gave little importance or priority to the improvement of the care of the insane. And so it was to remain for a considerable period.

The first world war intervened, as did the insurrection of 1916 and the war of independence. For the first time in fifty-one years there was a reduction in the mental hospital population. Despite the turbulent social background, the number of patients declined by an average of 578 annually during the years 1915 to 1918. To some extent the decline was influenced by the virulent epidemic of influenza of 1918 when there were 2,243 patient deaths from the illness. In Belfast asylum a fifth of the resident population died and about one in seven of all patients in Maryborough, Kilkenny, Armagh, and Castlebar asylums fell victim[26].

Emergence of the professional mental nurse

If little else changed in the asylum during the first few decades of the twentieth century there were important developments in the quality and status of its attendants. Since the care of the patient was to a considerable degree in the hands of the attendant this had a special significance.

In the past, as has been shown, one of the great deficiencies in the asylums lay in the nature of the caring staff. There was nothing about their work or their conditions likely to attract persons of merit even allowing for the assured weekly wage still difficult enough to find in many parts of Ireland. Physical height and strength had for long been the only essential requirements in their selection. The new committees of management saw no reason to change these criteria. Dr Drapes, the medical superintendent of Enniscorthy asylum, complained in 1902 'it is difficult to bring home to some minds, particularly those of very economic views, that the work of an asylum attendant is on quite a different level and very far removed from the work of an ordinary labourer'[27]. Each asylum committee settled its own conditions for its employers but there was little difference in approach. In Derry in 1910 the annual wages of male attendants varied between £20 and £25; females received £12; food, accommodation and uniform were also provided. Staff ratios continued to be kept extremely low. In Sligo at this period there was one male attendant to seventeen patients and one female to fifteen patients. The hours were long and little free time was given. On average, attendants worked eighty-three hours weekly[28].

The social standing of asylum workers could hardly be lower, something which the attitude of the asylum authorities did nothing to improve. A report commissioned by *The Lancet* during the 1870s had warned medical superintendents not to permit any of their own family to be involved in the work of the asylum. It pointed out that 'the circumstances of a superintendent's wife acting as matron involves a sacrifice of social position injurious, if not fatal, to success . . . indeed it is inconceivable that a man of position and culture would allow his family to have any connection with an asylum'[29]. It was a view echoed thirty years later when during 1907 the management committee of Sligo asylum discovered that the medical superintendent, Dr Gilcriest, had married the matron. Mr P. McHugh, MP, a member of the committee, declared vehemently that 'the duties discharged by the matron were such that no doctor's wife should be asked to do'. The committee asked Mrs Gilcriest to resign. She refused. Dr Gilcriest himself was then threatened with dismissal and asked to explain why he had not sought permission to marry the matron. After he insisted on his right to marry a wife of his choice both he and his wife were allowed to remain in their posts but only after considerable discussion by the committee[30].

In keeping with their generally unsympathetic attitude towards their employees managements were very reluctant to pay pensions when long-serving members retired. Before 1909 superannuation payments were entirely discretionary[31]. Pensions were not popular with public representatives who saw them as not only an unwarranted imposition on the taxpayer but as encouraging improvidence. Dr Nolan, the superintendent of Downpatrick asylum, described the heartsearching of his asylum committee when faced with an application for a pension:

> ... many inconsequent matters are raised in discussion and everything from the state of the country and the national debt to the problematical amount of the other possible sources of income of the individual concerned ... The fact that if he is reported to have savings often leads to the reduction of the pension[32].

By now, however, asylum workers were becoming organised in their own interests and their collective voice was beginning to be heard. Asylum doctors already had a mouthpiece for their views in the Irish branch of the Medico-Psychological Association but this was primarily a professional organisation and not to any serious degree a body that agitated for better working conditions. In 1895 the Asylum Workers Association was established in Britain mainly to promote the interests of nurses and attendants but some doctors and clerks also joined it. The association was open to Irish membership and by 1909 it had fewer than three hundred members drawn from eleven asylums[33]. It was a small response bearing in mind the extent of the Irish asylum system and its poor staff conditions, but opposition by hospital managements, including some medical superintendents, to anything that smacked of trade unionism was a major deterrent. In 1911 arising from the attitude of the management committee of the Richmond asylum the honorary secretary of the association wrote to the *Irish Times* assuring the public that there was 'no taint of trade unionism' in the constitution of the association [34].

One of the association's early achievements with the introduction in 1909 of guaranteed pensions to certain long-serving staff. Subsequent legislation provided further improvements[35]. This indication that organised workers could achieve some improvements in their conditions led to an increase in the association's Irish membership and, eventually, to the establishment of an independent Irish body for attendants. The new body was the Irish Asylum Attendants Executive set up in 1911 following a meeting convened by staff of Maryborough asylum [36]. Most asylums subsequently formed attendants' associations but as they had not the status, unity or strength of a trade union they achieved little. During the years of the 1914-18 war prices increased substantially but, in general, there was no improvement in the pay of asylum staff. Eventually, in October 1917, representatives of attendants from the majority of the asylums convened in the Trades Hall in Dublin and formed the Irish Asylum Workers Union[37].

The next six or seven years represented a period of trade union militancy in the asylums as the attendants agitated for better conditions. In Monaghan asylum in February 1919 the staff barricaded themselves into part of the asylum and raised a red flag on the roof. Here, surrounded by a force of 180 policemen and cheered on by the patients, they held out for several days until persuaded by a local clergyman to submit to an arbitration procedure[38]. In Clonmel later the same year a strike of attendants led to the 726 inmates being left in charge of four or five staff. Some of the patients escaped by swimming the Suir in which one of them was reported to have drowned. An attempt was made to burn down the residence of the medical superintendent. The strike lasted for several months[39]. Occasionally a strike was settled more quickly and with little formality. In Maryborough the staff walked out of the asylum in protest against low wages, after having locked all the patients into one building. Some of them broke out and went home. Andy Dunne, who was the asylum's tailor and a striker at the time, later recalled the event in a graphic manner:

> I had a patient working with me . . . Denny, said I,
> what happened to you to break out? 'I'll tell you the
> God's truth,' said he, 'I was afraid. They were throw-
> ing chairs and everything'. P.J. Meehan — he was the
> board's man and he followed us up the town. Said he
> 'for God's sake lads go back, I'll get you your wages,
> don't stay out and leave the patients there; I'll see
> that you get your rights'. That finished it. And P.J.
> Meehan did what he said. In 1921, nearly two years
> after the strike, I got four pound ten a week[40].

It was reasonably good pay by the standards of the times.
There is no doubt that the asylum staffs in general benefited
considerably during these years from the pressures of their
union.

Following the withdrawal of the British administration
from Ireland the new native government found itself beset
with economic difficulties during the 1920s. In some instances
local authorities were forced to reduce the pay of their
employees, including mental hospital staff. This gave rise to
strikes which were dealt with in a tough manner by the
managements. In 1924 when the committee of Letterkenny
District Mental Hospital abolished certain allowances all but
seven of the staff caring for 616 patients went on strike. The
committee, with the encouragement of the Minister for Local
Government and Public Health, immediately recruited new
staff to replace the strikers and 'normal conditions were
restored'[41].

By the 1940s it was clear to staffs that the fact that they
were then represented by a number of unions, had to negoti-
ate with individual hospital authorities, and that conditions
varied considerably between hospitals called for a more
unified approach. This culminated in most mental hospital
staffs joining the Irish Transport and General Workers Union
and to negotiations with the Minister for Health and county
managers in 1955 which led to parity of conditions between
all the district mental hospitals[42].

While trade union success in achieving improved pay and other conditions tended to advance the quality of staff recruited into the mental hospital service, their development as a trained body of nurses moved slowly. The extent to which hospital staffs availed themselves of the instruction provided under the aegis of the Medico-Psychological Association depended largely on the encouragement given by medical superintendents. Sometimes none was given. There was, in any event, little real inducement to an attendant to undertake the examinations since for a considerable period of time acquisition of a certificate meant an increase of only £2 annually in his wages. Furthermore the level of education of many of the attendants was such that they would hardly be capable of coping with an examination. In 1910 most of the attendant staff in Derry asylum held a certificate but this was quite exceptional for the period; in some asylums very few, if any, of the staff had a qualification[43]. Even as late as 1925 none of the staff in Ennis had undertaken the training course and only a small number of those in Carlow, Kilkenny, Clonmel and Killarney held certificates[44].

But the world of nursing was changing and would inevitably affect the mental hospitals as it had the general hospital system. Legislation of 1919 had established the General Nursing Council of Ireland (now replaced by An Bord Altranais) to standardise and supervise nurse training and to register those who qualified[45]. It hastened the end of the era of the untrained nurse and raised not only the quality but the status of those who undertook nursing. The council's register provided for different categories of nurses including those trained in the nursing and care of persons with mental diseases. Persons who already held the certificate of the Royal Medico-Psychological Association were granted automatic registration but after 1935 admission to the register had to be through the council's own examinations. Individual mental hospitals had to be recognised as suitable training centres before candidates were accepted for examination[46]. This requirement placed hospital managements under pressure to ensure that there were active programmes of care within their institutions.

Impetus was given to the training of the mental hospital staffs by the government commission that reported in 1927 on services for the sick and destitute poor. It recommended that eventually all the attendant staff in the hospitals should be trained nurses and that no one should be recruited unless capable of taking advantage of the instruction given[47].

The change over from hospitals staffed by untrained personnel to those having a full complement of professionally trained staff was a slow process and was completed only during the 1960s. As late as 1951 Dr Joseph Kearney, inspector of mental hospitals, reported that only half the members of the staff of the Kilkenny hospital were qualified in mental nursing[48]. Older attendants recruited on a basis that did not require them to undergo nursing examinations could not be compelled to undertake studies. Those who did so were not always popular with their colleagues since they were sometimes preferred for promotion. John Gill, a qualified nurse who worked in Portlaoise mental hospital (formerly Maryborough asylum) during and after the 1930s, later recalled:

> There was an awful lot of cutting and skelping — you had to keep a low profile in the set-up; as a matter of fact I never wore my medal — just for a quiet life[49].

Eventually the union insisted that every promotion should be on a seniority basis irrespective of whether the individual concerned was professionally qualified or not. It was an entirely staff-oriented view that disregarded the benefits to patients of trained staff particularly those in supervisory positions. It marked the beginning of a lengthy period of union recalcitrance and restrictive practices in relation to staff organisation and promotion. From being a poorly conditioned, voiceless and powerless worker the attendant of the lunatic asylum had now emerged as the mental (later psychiatric) nurse, a major, if not the dominant force, in the mental hospital system.

Under native government
With the departure of the British administration the Minister

for Local Government (later Local Government and Public Health) became responsible for public health services and the relief of the poor[50]. The poor law system of the previous regime was abolished; general hospitals and workhouses were re-organised into county systems consisting of county homes and county, district and fever hospitals; the mental hospital system remained basically unchanged at local level but its central direction became the responsibility of the minister. One of the inspectors of lunacy, Thomas Considine, retired and his colleague William Dawson was appointed to one of two similar posts under the Ministry of Home Affairs of the new Northern Ireland government. A single inspector of mental hospitals, Daniel Kelly, was appointed for the Irish Free State. Six of the district asylums, Antrim, Armagh, Belfast, Downpatrick, Derry and Omagh now passed to the northern administration[51]. Two of these asylums, Belfast and Derry, were then being gradually replaced by new buildings at other sites. In the Irish Free State references to lunacy, lunatics and asylums disappeared from the official nomenclature; statutory sanction was given in 1925 to the change of name from lunatic asylum to mental hospital[52].

There was little public discussion during the 1920s on the mental hospital services. They were hard times politically and economically. Ernest Blythe, Minister for Local Government, conceded in 1923 that some of the mental hospitals were seriously short of finance but blamed it on the failure of ratepayers to pay their rates[53]. Reference has already been made to mental hospital committees reducing the pay of their staff. There was overcrowding and understaffing; medical superintendents were so overwhelmed with administrative duties that they had little time to attend the patients[54]. During 1925 the government established a commission to look critically at the laws and administration relating to the provisions for the sick and destitute poor in general. It was asked specifically to examine the position of the mentally ill and the mentally handicapped. In the course of their work the commissioners visited almost all the institutions in the country and their report contains a good account of the various services of the period[55].

The general picture that emerged from many of the district mental hospitals was one of considerable overcrowding and inactivity with regimens that appeared to be based on apathy or pessimism or a combination of both. Many of the criticisms struck a familiar note; *plus ça change, plus c'est la même chose*. In a few places, notably in Carlow, a considerable effort had been made to create a bright and cheerful atmosphere; but they were exceptional:

> ... in most of the institutions the impression was not so favourable. . . . The drab and cheerless appearance of the wards, the neglect to remedy small defects; the untidy state of the grounds, the large number of idle patients which was noticeable in some establishments were in some degree indicative of a failure of administration. Some of the arrangements we saw left us under the impression that the routine of institutional life would need to be re-surveyed from the point of view of the patients' comfort. In one hospital the shutters of the dormitories were closed shortly after five o'clock on a summer afternoon, preparatory to patients going to bed at seven o'clock. Even when empty these dormitories were stuffy and must become almost intolerable on a summer night. In several the patients dress and undress in the corridors and on the stairways, and in one actually come into the dormitories without any clothes. This practice seems to have originated as a measure of precaution, but we find it is a precaution that it is not found necessary to adopt everywhere and is one which must affront the sense of decency of many patients[56].

If the mental hospital scene was unchanged and unchanging little better could be said about the position of the 1,900 largely imbecile and idiot patients then accommodated in the former workhouses now somewhat euphemistically termed county homes. The report commented: 'their condition . . .

shows no improvement; it is, we consider, on the whole worse by reason of congregating in one county home the insane inmates of several workhouses'[57]. The report found little progress in providing special facilities for idiot and imbecile children. One new institution had opened for Catholic children. It was St Vincent's Home at Cabra in County Dublin, established by the Sisters of Charity of St Vincent de Paul in 1926 in an old workhouse school. The only other special centre, Stewart's Institution, now had a population that consisted entirely of adults who had been admitted there as children. The original idea of training had, according to a witness, 'entirely disappeared during the last twenty years and Stewart's Institution is an asylum for the most hopeless cases'[58].

If the state of affairs that confronted the commissioners has a familiar ring so, too, had some of its recommendations. Its main proposals echoed Bishop Kelly's views of twenty years earlier: that there should be a system of auxiliary mental hospitals established in old workhouses to relieve in an economical manner the pressure in the existing district mental hospitals and to provide for the insane then in the county homes. The auxiliaries would be superintended by a matron, there would be no resident doctor and, as the patients would not be violent or dangerous, the staff could be entirely female[59]. While it recommended that local authorities be enabled to assist parents financially in sending their handicapped children for training to an approved institution it expressed no views about the manner of further development of such a service even though it was then, effectively, limited to one institution, St Vincent's.

In some respects the views of the commission were very progressive. Impressed by Scottish experience it recommended the introduction of outpatient services for the mentally ill as well as the treatment in a general hospital setting of certain short-term patients[60]. It also drew attention to the fact that the majority of patients were still being admitted under statutory provisions that labelled them 'dangerous lunatics' when their actual condition was sometimes described in such mild terms as 'wandering' or 'talking incoherently'. It recommended the repeal of all existing lunacy laws and the introduction of new and simpler procedures for admission, including voluntary admission, which would safeguard the rights of the patient[61].

But there was little chance of early action on the commission's proposals for any of the mentally abnormal. They represented only a small segment of a wide range of recommendations which dealt with all aspects of the provisions for the sick and disadvantaged poor. The report was particularly critical of the facilities and standards of care in many of the general hospitals and found various instances of discrimination against the sick poor. Ireland was still haunted by the former workhouse system. There were grievous shortcomings in provisions for the old and infirm, for the tubercular, for unmarried mothers and their children, for the orphan and deserted child. Set against the needs of some of these groups the claims for the mentally afflicted could not be seen, and were not seen, to command a special urgency or priority.

The Walls Come Tumbling Down

Economically the 1930s, the war and immediate post-war years were difficult times unfavourable to social advances. The main thrust of government policies was towards industrial development, creating additional employment and stemming emigration. In the circumstances it is unlikely that resources of any significance would have been available to improve any aspect of the hospital system without the initiation of the Irish Hospitals Sweepstakes. It would be difficult, in the event, to exaggerate the importance of the sweepstakes to Irish public hospitals over the subsequent thirty years. Apart from the mental hospitals, the stock of institutions at the beginning of that period was largely rooted in voluntary hospitals of eighteenth and early nineteenth century origins, and in the workhouses of the 1840s. It required a huge investment to create a system based on twentieth century concepts of care; the extent to which it was achieved was due in large measure to the earnings of the sweepstakes.

The profits of the sweepstakes were originally intended for distribution only among a group of voluntary hospitals. The monies were statutorily taken over in 1931 by the Minister for Local Government and Public Health and under the new, and subsequent amending, provisions local authority as well as voluntary hospitals became eligible for grants[1]. Public policy favoured general hospital development and, in a situation where many persons were dying from tuberculosis, the opening of new sanatoria. In consequence there were impor-

191

tant additions and improvements to these categories of institutions, in particular between the mid-30s and the mid-50s.

The district mental hospitals benefited, but to a considerably lesser degree. A new hospital to serve County Louth was opened in Ardee in 1933; Ballinasloe was given the support of a branch hospital, Castlerea, Co. Roscommon, in 1940[2]. The cost of replacing any of the old mental hospitals would have been daunting and in general the aim was to soften some of their harsher features. Compared with the sums spent on the other categories of hospital the expenditure was extremely limited. Between 1931 and 1955 less than £1.5 million was allocated to mental hospitals from sweepstake funds out of a total distribution of £35 million[3]. Furthermore it is questionable whether the expenditure of relatively small sums in an attempt to improve the spartan standards of nineteenth century buildings achieved anything worthwhile. In 1960 Vincent Dolphin, inspector of mental hospitals, pointed to the 'uphill struggle' involved in trying to modernise the hospitals[4].

Improved services for mentally handicapped
The period was, therefore, not notable for improvements to the physical fabric of the existing mental hospitals but it marked, nevertheless, the practical recognition by the government of the need for extra provisions for mentally handicapped persons. During these years about £1.25 million from sweepstake funds were used for the creation of new residential centres for the mentally handicapped mainly to accommodate children[5]. In time these centres would contribute to the gradual reduction in mental hospital populations.

A distinguishing feature of this newly developing service was that almost all the centres were operated by Catholic religious bodies which in some instances contributed substantially to the cost of their development. It was generally accepted that the difficult nature of the care involved would benefit by the vocational commitment of religious communities. There was also the consideration that some of the bodies concerned already had a considerable background of experience in looking after the mentally handicapped whereas the statutory health agencies had none. The Daughters of Charity, founded in the seventeenth century by Vincent de Paul, had a long tradition in this area. Their founder had been one of the first persons to attempt the education of idiots. The Brothers of Charity, of early nineteenth century Belgian origin, had experience of caring for the mentally abnormal in various parts of the world[6]. The Brothers of St John of God, also, were involved in many places abroad in this type of service. Their sixteenth century founder, John Cidade, had himself once been locked up as a madman and had been one of the first to treat mental illness as a sickness and not as a punishment for sin[7].

Four of the new centres were opened by the Daughters of Charity namely, St Joseph's, Clonsilla, Co. Dublin; the Hospital of the Holy Angels, Glenmaroon, Co. Dublin; St Vincent's, Lisnagry, Co. Limerick and St Theresa's, Blackrock, Co. Dublin. Three were developed under the aegis of the Brothers of St John of God — St Augustine's, Blackrock, Co. Dublin; St Mary's, Drumcar, Co. Louth; and St Raphael's, Celbridge, Co. Kildare and two under the Brothers of Charity — Our Lady of Good Counsel, Lota, Co. Cork and St Joseph's, Kilcornan, Co. Galway. The Sisters of La Sagesse established a centre at Cregg House, Co. Sligo and the Sisters of Jesus and Mary opened St Mary's, Delvin, Co. Westmeath. Most of these developments took place during the 1950s and were considerably added to in later years[8].

In architectural and operational terms there was an avoidance of the characteristics of the monolithic Victorian institution. In general the centres were planned as a complex of small single-storey buildings which recognised the needs of the different degrees of severity of mental handicap and facilitated a regimen of social training, physical activation, and occupational habilitation. Education was provided for the educable. While the centres were still institutional in character and not planned, as in later years, to simulate a home life, they were a far cry from the conditions which the idiots and the imbeciles of the past had endured.

A report prepared in 1943 by Dr Louis Clifford at the request of the Hospitals Commission had served as a stimulus to the provision of the additional facilities[9]. The Commission was a statutory body responsible for advising the Minister for Local Government and Public Health on the disbursement of the sweepstake funds. It had asked Clifford to carry out a survey on the incidence of mental handicap; this he did with a small team which examined several thousand children attending primary schools in selected city and rural areas. The findings were extrapolated to the population as a whole. Clifford concluded that there were altogether 66,000 mentally handicapped persons in the country of whom 21,000 were children. In the light of more recent investigations these figures were grossly over-estimated. His calculations would have meant that there were twenty-two mentally handicapped persons for every thousand of the population compared with a later 1974 estimate of approximately eight per thousand[10].

The criteria and methods used for ascertaining handicap in the two studies were different and, in any event, Clifford and his team had to work under severe limitations and difficulties. Because of the large number of children involved some of the tests of intelligence were administered in groups. Sometimes the teachers resented the disturbance of the school routine; many parents were unco-operative; an investigation of this sort was patently unwelcome particularly in rural areas. Clifford's report gives a picture of the taboos and attitudes connected with mental deficiency in Ireland in the early 1940s. Having a mentally handicapped child was widely seen by parents as a disgrace and a reflection on the family. It was especially resented by the higher social strata; those in the lower social groups were more philosophical about their misfortune. Handicapped children were sometimes hidden away in top rooms and seldom taken out except at night. Sometimes those attending school were kept away from it on the day of Clifford's investigation so that they would not be identified as handicapped. This was not a deterrent to Clifford who pursued his work with notable determination. Absentee children were visited in their homes; some fled and were pursued by him through the fields so that they could be brought for examination. At times the investigators found that children in rural schools who *prima facie* appeared intellectually deficient were backward simply because their parents discouraged academic achievement. They feared that a child who did well at school might eventually head for a city career and be a consequent loss to them on the land. Crushed between the academic demands of the school and the hostile attitudes of the parents some children showed signs of emotional disturbance.

Until 1957 the developing services for mentally handicapped persons were based almost entirely on residential centres; subsequently care, education and, in some instances, sheltered employment were provided in an increasing number of day centres. In Dublin, St Michael's House, and in Cork, the Cork Polio and General After-Care Association began providing a large range of day educational and care facilities. In other parts of the country the day centres were operated mainly by voluntary groups of parents and friends of mentally handicapped persons[11].

Changes in mental treatment laws

With the passage of time the need to change the outdated mental hospital admission laws of 1867 became more obvious. More liberal provisions inaugurated in the United Kingdom in 1930 had been extended to Northern Ireland in 1932[12]. They introduced voluntary admissions and a procedure for the reception of other patients on a temporary basis following an application by a relative. It was not, however, until 1944 that Dr Con Ward, parliamentary secretary to Sean MacEntee, the Minister for Local Government and Public Health, introduced in Dail Eireann proposals for changes which eventually became the Mental Treatment Act, 1945. The fact that a separate minister for health was created shortly afterwards in 1947 helped to strengthen the central administration and implementation of the new laws[13]. They contained radical reforms and are a landmark in Irish social

legislation. All the earlier unrepealed lunacy laws, except
those relating to criminal lunatics and wards of court, were
replaced by provisions detailed in almost three hundred
sections of the Act. The new measure might be faulted for its
prolixity and, in particular, for the welter of bureaucratic
classifications and procedures introduced in relation to the
admission of patients. But its basic principles were admirably
enlightened.

Its most important features were the admission and discharge procedures. They departed entirely from the long-
standing process already described whereby most patients
were committed on the order of two peace commissioners
(previously justices of the peace). Under the new arrangements,
based entirely on medical certification, a person could be
admitted to a mental hospital either as a voluntary or a
detained patient. Voluntary admissions required the minimum
of formality. Detained patients fell into two categories:
temporary patients and 'persons of unsound mind'. Temporary
patients were those who in the medical view required up to
six months' treatment and were considered unsuitable to be
voluntary patients. Persons of unsound mind could be detained
indefinitely[14]. A legal obligation was imposed on the hospital
authorities to discharge a recovered patient. Various other
patient safeguards were provided for, including the appointment of visiting committees to the hospitals; the right of a
relative or friend to appeal to the minister for the discharge
of the patient; and the right of any person to apply to the
minister to have the patient examined by independent
medical practitioners[15]. In addition the inspector of mental
hospitals was given special powers and duties to ensure that
there was no abuse of the detention arrangements[16].

These changes in the law helped to place the mental hospital
in a new perspective. The fact that many patients were now
free to enter or to leave whenever they wished, started the
demolition of the physical and attitudinal barriers that had
surrounded it for so long. Furthermore, the more liberal
admission and discharge processes could hardly have come at
a more propitious time, for there were other events taking

place in the management of mental illness which would eventually hasten the end of isolation and help to bring the walls tumbling down.

The new therapies

The 1930s and 1940s saw the origin of new scientific ideas and discoveries which transformed psychiatry, created new hope for the patients and their friends and hastened the demise of the traditional mental hospital. Psychotherapy, requiring the establishment of a close therapist-patient relationship, developed as a method of understanding and correcting the distorted communicating process of the psychotic patient. Fundamentally it differed little from the earlier concept of moral treatment but it had the advantage that the therapist now started with a greater understanding of the workings of the human mind. There had been, however, a hope for a long time that an effective physical method of treatment would be discovered. There was a step in this direction during the 1930s when analeptic drugs were used to induce convulsions in schizophrenic patients. Towards the end of the decade a more refined and safer form of convulsive treatment — electro-convulsive therapy — was introduced and became widely regarded as beneficial particularly in its anti-depressant effects. The treatment of schizophrenia by insulin also dates from the same period; but enthusiasm for it was fading by the end of the 1950s when it was becoming clear that the benefits claimed for the method had as much to do with the intensive medical and nursing care required as with the drug itself. In the 1940s and 1950s leucotomy, a technique involving surgery of the brain, was resorted to in some hospitals when other strategies failed. It was found to be hazardous and unpredictable and is now rarely used. The greatest advance came, however, with the development in the early 1950s of the chlorpromazine group of drugs. They had a major impact on the treatment of schizophrenia and other serious psychotic conditions; by enabling patients to adopt a relaxed mood there was an immediate reduction in the intensity of disturbed behaviour. A few years later the introduction

197

of anti-depressant drugs, notably imipramine and amitripty-
line, proved to be an effective means of treating depression[17].

The new chemotherapy did not, it was soon discovered,
provide lasting cures; but it would be difficult, nevertheless,
to exaggerate its influence on the methods and organisation
of the mental treatment services. It was now possible to consider alternatives to the deeply rooted policy of isolation and
confinement. The belief that it was wrong to confine all
categories of insane patients in large security conscious hospitals had been around for a long time. Many years previously
Maudsley had defined insanity as 'a want of harmony ...
between the individual and his social medium by reason of
some defect or fault of mind in him as prevents him living
and working among his kind in the social organisation'[18].
The correction of this disharmony in the isolation of a mental
hospital obviously posed difficulties since the setting was an
abnormal one. As already described, enlightened doctors, such
as Connolly Norman as early as the turn of the century, had
pointed to the logical alternative: that there should be greater
emphasis on the non-institutional management of insanity.
As the twentieth century progressed and psychiatry became
more scientifically based there was greater support for this
view. But those who introduced more liberal regimens had
substantial obstacles to overcome. The public-at-large continued to see the mentally ill person in terms of socially
unacceptable behaviour: unpredictable and potentially
dangerous. There was a reluctance to accept that care could
be provided for such a person in a manner other than within
the controls of the traditional mental hospital.

The new drugs removed much of the justification for such
attitudes. Under their influence patients within the hospitals
were able to function in a more acceptable and controlled
way; more important, many could avoid hospital admission
or return home earlier. Almost overnight the more depressing
sights and sounds of the day rooms disappeared; doors were
opened, gates were unlocked. This 'open-door' policy shifted
the emphasis away from residential care and from the mental
hospital itself. More symbolically the walls started coming

down. At Carlow district mental hospital, for instance, the resident medical superintendent, Bertram Blake, with the support of the management committee, had the high surrounding walls reduced to about three feet and topped with flowers. Some local people protested and fitted locks to their doors; but their concern was of short duration[19]. Blake and other progressive psychiatrists like him were able to show that the disappearance of locks and walls offered no threat to the populace.

Out-patient clinics increased in number and attendance; the first day hospitals, rehabilitation workshops and hostels aimed at helping patients to return to the community appeared. Earlier changes in entitlement to free health services had removed the long-time pauper associations of the mental hospital by placing it on the same basis as other hospitals and broadening eligibility for care[20]. By 1961 more patients were being treated at out-patient clinics than within the hospitals and, by the end of the following year, almost sixty per cent of the in-patient admissions were on a voluntary basis[21]. Coincidentally the sanatoria were closing because the treatment of tuberculosis had, too, been transformed by new chemotherapy. Between 1959 and 1966 large sanatoria at Ballyowen, Co. Dublin; Heatherside, Co. Cork; Newcastle, Co. Wicklow; Crooksling, Co. Dublin, and various small centres were taken over by the mental treatment services to relieve the overcrowding in some of the old hospitals[22]. The Newcastle institution was eventually designated the district mental hospital for County Wicklow. Elsewhere, but not yet in Ireland, the practical integration of the treatment of physical and mental illness was under way. Government plans in the USA and the United Kingdom in the early 1960s provided for psychiatric units within general hospitals[23]. There was considerable support for views propounded by Professor Thomas McKeown of Birmingham University that the ideal hospital should be a single complex planned to meet the total sickness needs, physical and mental, of the community it served[24].

A gradual decline developed in the mental hospital population which had reached a peak of 21,075 in 1958[25]. It was steady but slow; thousands of those who had been long-term patients before the new era of psychiatry had gone beyond the stage of ever returning to the world outside the walls. It had, in any event, abandoned them, for many were unvisited by friend or relative. At the end of March 1963, forty-one per cent of the 19,800 patients then in the hospitals had been resident there for eighteen years or more. For eleven per cent of them the mental hospital had been their home for over twenty-eight years[26].

Incidence of mental illness

While the early 1960s was a period of great optimism for the treatment of mental illness in Ireland its incidence appeared to remain remarkably high compared with elsewhere. It is not appropriate to this broad historical study to investigate in depth the reasons why or to attempt an examination of a complex and specialised area. The salient facts are, however, relevant to the completion of the historical picture and call for some comment. The past indications of a high rate of Irish mental illness were confirmed by Walsh in 1963 in the first detailed study of hospital populations; there was further confirmation in a subsequent study[27]. They showed that between 1963 and 1978 the hospitalisation rate in Ireland remained about two and a half times the figure for English mental hospitals. Further studies into the causes of admission identified schizophrenia as the principal diagnosis while the number of cases of alcoholism annually was shown to be rapidly increasing. A striking feature of these studies was the high rate of illness among unmarried persons of both sexes, notably males. Even after allowing for the fact that some of the patients were congenitally abnormal and unlikely ever to marry the figure was remarkably high. Furthermore, an exceptionally large proportion of the male patients over this period consisted of unmarried farmers and farm labourers[28]. Abroad, too, admissions to psychiatric hospitals among Irish immigrants continued to be comparatively high as Dean and others showed in a study in relation to south-east England in

1976[29].

Because of the nature of mental illness and the absence of scientific certainties about the origins of some of its more serious forms it is impossible authoritatively to explain the reasons for these exceptional characteristics of the pattern of Irish insanity. It is possible now only to speculate why the past has left such an unwelcome heritage. The tendency to higher rates of mental illness among immigrant groups in general has already been described. A separate answer is required as to why the rate of mental illness in the resident population of Ireland appears to be comparatively high. There is almost certainly no single explanation. Apart from a few limited studies the comparative statistics of mental illness in different countries are based on hospital admissions and not on the total number of persons identified as being mentally ill. Thus persons receiving treatment outside of the hospital will not be included in the statistics. Some persons under care for mental disturbance will not even come within the ambit of the psychiatric services. For these reasons a country's standing in the comparative statistics of mental illness tends to be determined by the extent to which national policy bases its approach to treatment on admission to psychiatric hospitals or units.

On the face of it Ireland is hospital prone. In 1961 the Irish provision of 7.3 psychiatric beds per 1,000 population appeared to be the highest in the world[30]. While this figure has been reduced considerably in the interim period the latest available figure of 4.9 beds per 1,000 is still relatively high compared with other countries[31]. The high usage of beds in Ireland is also reflected in comparative figures of patient admissions. In 1981 the rate of admission of male patients in Ireland was almost three times that of English males. Where females were concerned the admission rate was almost twice that of England[32].

There is, it is suggested, a number of factors contributing to that situation. One is the historic fact that for a considerable period those in need of treatment or care for any disability in Ireland had little choice but to seek it within an institution.

In Britain, by comparison, the Elizabethan poor law provisions established a system of parochial charity which contained a considerable element of non-institutional care for the destitute, the sick and the infirm[33]. Thus, a tradition was established which carried over to later poor law developments and to the welfare state. Ireland did not have this parochial system. It had few social provisions of any sort until the nineteenth century. Neither the early nineteenth century voluntary dispensaries nor the later formal dispensary system established under poor law legislation in 1851[34] was capable of caring for other than the acutely ill. Furthermore the dispensary doctors were poorly paid, a position that continued until the system was replaced in 1972 by a 'choice-of-doctor' service, and they had no incentive to take on the care of burdensome patients. In any event, it would have been impossible, particularly in scattered rural areas, for a doctor working alone to assume any significant degree of responsibility for the long-term ill in his area.

The result was that when the nineteenth century workhouses and asylums were established they instantly became, as already described, receptacles for a whole range of human infirmity and deprivation. The fact that their services were widely availed of represented an ambivalent public attitude. On the one hand, admission to either category of institution was seen as carrying a stigma; on the other hand it was reluctantly acceptable to many people as the only answer to a whole range of social problems. This practice, facilitated by liberal admission procedures, continued as the nineteenth century institutions became the county homes, county hospitals, district hospitals and mental hospitals of the present century.

Furthermore, institutionalisation both under the British administration and, until recent times, under native government was regarded by the authorities as the most economic and controllable way of dealing with social problems. In any event, the remoteness of many of the rural population, bad communications and poor living standards were important considerations tending to favour a policy of bringing under one large roof those who needed care. Thus, the institution as a means of dealing with illness or infirmity in any form became a deeply rooted Irish practice which still leaves its influence despite the modern development of alternative methods of care. It is also an important element in the Irish economy. The local institution in many small Irish towns is not only a very assured centre of employment but a valuable consumer of goods produced and sold locally. In particular, district mental hospitals, because of their size, are seen as important economic units. Proposals to close hospitals, or parts of hospitals, of any category invariably arouse considerable local opposition and political controversy.

This deeply rooted attachment to local institutions obviously has implications for the manner in which patients are cared for since it is an influence on the extent to which new methods are adopted. It is clear from official reports that there is a considerable variation between health board areas as to the extent to which efforts are being made to provide alternatives to mental hospital admission[35]. The provision of day facilities, out-patient clinics, hostels and rehabilitation workshops show varying degrees of commitment. This is reflected in wide disparities in the rates of hospital admissions[36]. In one health board area, for instance, admissions during 1982 were at the rate of 702 per 100,000 population. In another area the corresponding figure was 1,147. The disparity cannot be explained in terms of demographic variations nor is there any evidence of differences in the extent or nature of mental illness between the areas.

The evidence clearly suggests that what contemporary Ireland has inherited is not a high level of mental illness but an excessive commitment to the mental hospital and the mental hospital bed. There may be other influences contributing to the unfavourable Irish statistics but they are likely to be marginal.

Nevertheless, the changes that have taken place over the last few decades have opened up a new period of hope and understanding for all who are mentally afflicted. Some of the progress has come from scientific advance; some from changes in the human heart. In many respects social prejudices rooted in centuries of malevolence and ignorance have diminished. Greater understanding has developed not only for the mentally ill and the mentally handicapped; there has been, for instance, a gradual acceptance of the illegitimate child and its mother. In the cavalcade of human history the lunatic and the bastard have long stood out as representing the constantly reviled, the universally rejected, the favoured terms of opprobrium. Now as the twentieth century moves towards its end all countries where freedom and civilised thinking prevail are rejecting the age-old injustices towards both of them.

It has taken a long time.

Epilogue

Separate government commissions of enquiry on mental handicap and mental illness reported in 1965 and 1966 respectively[1]. Their main recommendations reflected developments elsewhere some of which were already under way in Ireland. The commission on mental illness proposed wide-ranging provisions for non-institutional treatment and community support and favoured the inclusion of short-term psychiatric units in general hospitals. The commission on mental handicap recommended that residential services for the handicapped should continue to be based mainly on religious and voluntary groups. Emphasis was given to the establishment of care and educational services on a day basis. A firm terminology was proposed and adopted, viz. *mentally handicapped* persons, classified according to intelligence quotient. The words 'idiot' and 'imbecile' now disappeared from official use.

To a large extent the services developed along the lines recommended. The establishment of eight health boards in 1970 to take over the operation of the health services in general from the local authorities facilitated improvements in the whole health area[2]. A broad network of services for the mentally ill was created outside the hospital. They included a community psychiatric nursing service involving home visiting by nurses based on the local mental hospital. Psychiatric units became a feature of most of the larger general hospitals. Attendances at outpatient services increased but so, too, did

205

hospital admissions; many of them were re-admissions. Shorter duration of stay in hospital meant, however, that by the end of 1983 the total mental hospital population had fallen to 12,802[3]. A study group reporting to the Minister for Health at the end of 1984 recommended the further extension of community based services and the development of the long-term goal of treating all admissions in the psychiatric units of general hospitals[4]. It envisaged a continuing reduction in the number of long-stay patients and urged that the main thrust of psychiatric policy should be to move away from the large traditional style mental hospital. New mental legislation enacted in 1981, but not implemented up to early 1986, would have the effect of further advancing the integration of the care of mentally ill and physically ill persons and provide new safeguards for the small number of persons subject to compulsory care[5].

Residential accommodation and day facilities for mentally handicapped persons expanded considerably from the 1960s onwards. Increasing attention was given to 'normalisation', viz. the creation of a living and training environment likely to advance the integration of the handicapped persons into normal society. This led to a considerable change in the character of residential care which now aims as far as possible to reflect a family setting. At the end of 1982 about 9,000 mentally handicapped adults and children were being cared for in special residential and day care centres of whom 6,250 were being looked after on a residential basis[6]. The religious and voluntary bodies already working in this area were joined by many others, notably, the Camphill Village Community, the Irish Sisters of Charity, the Rosminian Fathers, Western Care, Cheeverstown House, the Franciscan Missionaries of the Divine Motherhood and various local groups consisting largely of parents and friends of mentally handicapped persons. In some instances health boards established residential centres of their own in the absence of suitable voluntary organisations.

Ireland's admission to the European Economic Community in 1973 gave access to financial support from the European Social Fund thus enabling considerable improvements in services for the vocational training and social integration of mentally handicapped and long-term mentally ill persons. Furthermore greater public concern and sympathy for them were stimulated by the efforts of the Mental Health Association and the National Association for the Mentally Handicapped and by the work of small self-help groups such as the Schizophrenia Association and the Society for Autistic Children.

Early in 1986 Barry Desmond, the Minister for Health, announced the government's intention to close the district mental hospitals at Carlow and Castlerea. This step was in keeping with the policy suggested in the report of 1984. It marked the beginning of a new era in the care of the mentally ill in Ireland[7].

Bibliography

List of Abbreviations

Comms. jn. Ire.   Journals of the Irish House of Commons.
H.C.   House of Commons papers.
ILI   Inspectors of Lunatics in Ireland.
ILNI   Inspectors of Lunacy, Northern Ireland.
IMH   Inspector of Mental Hospitals.
JSSISI   Journal of the Statistical and Social Inquiry
                  Society of Ireland.
O.P.   Official Papers (State Paper Office).

Manuscript and Unpublished Sources

Bloomfield Hospital: small quantity of papers re meetings and appeals. Society of Friends Library Dublin.

Burke Joseph, Assistant Poor Law Commissioner correspondence books 1838-1854. Public Record Office.

Chief Secretary's Office: official papers 1790-1922 and registered papers 1818-1924. State Paper Office Dublin.

Clifford Dr L.S.: report to Hospitals Commission of investigation of mental deficiency and sane epilepsy in Ireland May 1943.

Folklore archives: University College Dublin.

Larcom Papers, National Library Dublin.

Mayo Papers, National Library Dublin.

Monteagle Papers, National Library Dublin.

Murphy Daniel: unpublished historical account of psychiatric nurse staff, Our Lady's Hospital, Cork 1851-1955.

Office of Lunatic Asylums: Dublin Castle: a few miscellaneous papers 1882-1891. Department of Health Dublin.

St Patrick's Hospital, Dublin: Board minutes August 1746 to September 1835 (in the Hospital).

Stewart's Institution: Minute book of sub-committee 1868-1870 and miscellaneous reports. Stewart's Hospital.

Books, Articles, Pamphlets

Abraham George Whitley, *The law and practice of lunacy in Ireland.* Dublin 1886.

Achmet, *A report on the cases relieved and cured in the baths appropriated for the reception of the poor.* Dublin 1777.

Anon, *Five letters on the subject of the poor of Ireland* 1816.

Apley John ed., *Care of the Handicapped child.* Suffolk 1978.

Archdall Mervyn, *Monasticon Hibernicum.* London 1986.

Association for the Suppression of Mendicity in Dublin, *Tenth report of the General Committee.* Dublin 1827.

Ball Elrington, *The Correspondence of Jonathan Swift,* 5 vol. London 1910.

Banks J.T., The writ *'de lunatico inquirendo'* in the case of Jonathan Swift D.D., Dean of St Patrick's with observations 1861 in *Dublin Quarterly Journal of Medical Science* xxxi.

Biddiss Michael D. ed., *Images of Race.* Leicester 1979.

Binchy D.A., Bretha Crolige in *Eriú* xii.

Blake John A., *Defects in the Moral Treatment of Insanity in the Public Lunatic Asylums of Ireland.* Dublin 1862.

Blumer G. Alder and Richardson A.B. eds., *Commitment, Detention, Care and Treatment of the Insane* (report of international congress Chicago 1893). New York 1894.

Bonner Brian, *Our Inis Eoghain Heritage.* Dublin 1972.

Bowen Desmond, *The Protestant Crusade in Ireland 1800-1870.* Dublin 1978.

Boyd-Barrett Edward, Modern Psychotherapy and Our Asylums in *Studies* xii, 1924.

Brewer J.S. and Bullen William eds. *Calendar of the Carew*

Manuscripts, 6 vol. London 1867-1873.

Burdett Henry C., *Hospitals and Asylums of the World* 4 vol. London 1891.

Burton Robert (Democritus Junior), *The Anatomy of Melancholy,* 2 vol. London 1806.

Brooks Eric St John. *Register of St John the Baptist without the New Gate Dublin.* Dublin 1936.

Byrd Max, *Visits to Bedlam.* Columbia 1974.

Camden William, *Britannia* trans. Edward Gibson. London 1695.

Carr John, *The Stranger in Ireland 1805.* London 1806.

Carstairs G.M. and Kennedy P.F., *Social Science in relation to Psychiatry in Companion to Psychiatric Studies.* sec. ed. 1978. London.

Carte Thomas, *A History of the life of James Duke of Ormonde 1610-8,* 3 vol. 1736.

Carte Thomas, *The Life of the Duke of Ormond.* new ed., 6 vol. Oxford 1851.

Census of Ireland 1851: part three, report on the status of disease. Dublin 1854.

Chadwick Nora K., Geilt in *Scottish Gaelic Studies* v, pt. 2. 1942.

Chafetz Morris and Demone Harold W., *Alcholism and Society.* New York 1962.

Chatterton Lady Henrietta, *Rambles in the South of Ireland during the year 1838.* 2 vol. London 1839.

Cohn Norman, *Europes Inner Demons.* London 1839.

Collins John, The Evolution of County Government in *Administration* i (2), 1953.

Cooney John, *A Service for the Mentally Handicapped.* Dublin 1961.

Conellan Owen, trans, *The Annals of Ireland translated from the original Irish of the Four Masters.* Dublin 1846.

Cork Historical and Archaeological Society, *Journal* vii, second series, 1902.

Corbett William J., On the statistics of insanity past and present in JSSISI vi, 1871-6.

Craft Michael ed., *Tredgold's Mental Retardation*, 12th ed. London 1979.

Craik Henry, *The Life of Jonathan Swift*, 2 vol. London 1894.

Croker T. Crofton, *Researches in the South of Ireland*. London 1824.

Cummins N. Marshall, *Some chapters of Cork medical history*. Cork 1957.

Cytryn Leon and Reginald S. Lourie, Mental Retardation in *Comprehensive Textbook of Psychiatry* 1967.

Davis Herbert ed., *Swift — Poetical Works*. London 1967.

Davies Lloyd, Why are People so Cruel? in *World Health* April 1983.

Dean Geoffrey, Downing Helen, Shelley Emer, First Admissions by Psychiatric Hospitals in south east England in 1976 among immigrants from Ireland in *British Medical Journal* cclxxxii, June 1981.

Dictionary of National Biography, 22 vol. London 1909.

Donnelly James S., *The land and the people of nineteenth century Cork*. London 1975.

Drapes Thomas, *On the alleged increase of insanity in Ireland, 1894*.

Eachard Laurence, *An Exact Description of Ireland*. London 1691.

Earl of Orrery John, *Remarks on the life and Writings of Dr Jonathan Swift*. Dublin 1757.

Ehrenpreis Irvin, *Swift: the Man, his Works and the Age*. London 1962.

Ellis Henry ed., *Original letters illustrative of English history*, third series, iv. London 1846.

Fallows Marjorie R., *Irish Americans: Identity and Assimilation*. New Jersey 1979.

Finnane Mark, *Insanity and the Insane in Post-Famine Ireland*. London 1981.

Fitzgerald P. and McGregor J.J., *The History, Topography and Antiquities of the County and City of Limerick*, 2 vol. London 1826.

Fitzpatrick Jeremiah, *An Essay on Gaol Abuses and Means*

of Redressing them. Dublin 1784.

Forestor Thomas trans., *The Historical Works of Giraldus Cambrensis.* London 1905.

Foster Edward, *A letter to Sydenham Singleton, chairman of committee . . . to enquire into the state of lunatics in this city.* Dublin 1777.

Foucault Michel, *Discipline and Punish: The Birth of the Prison,* trans. Alan Sheridan. London 1977.

Fownes William, *Methods proposed for regulating the poor supporting of some and employing others according to their several capacities.* Dublin 1725.

Freedman Alfred and others, *Comprehensive Textbook of Psychiatry,* 2 vol. Baltimore 1975.

Freeman Hugh, *Trends in the Mental Health Services.* Oxford 1963.

Fry Elizabeth and Gurney Joseph John, *Report addressed to the Marquess Wellesley, Lord Lieutenant.* London 1827.

Gelder Michael and others, *Textbook of Psychiatry.* Oxford 1983.

General rules and regulations for the management of district lunatic asylums in Ireland. Dublin 1894.

Gilbert J.T. and Rosa M. eds., *Calendar of Ancient Records of Dublin,* 17 vol. Dublin 1889-1916.

Goodwin Donald and Samuel B. Guze, *Psychiatric Diagnosis* sec. ed. Oxford 1979.

Granville J.M., *Care and Cure of Insane,* 2 vols. 1877.

Gwynn Aubrey and Hadcock R. Neville, *Medieval Religious Houses in Ireland.* London 1970.

Gwynn Stephen, *The Life and Friendships of Dean Swift.* London 1933.

Hallaran William Saunders, *Practical Observations on the Causes and Cure of Insanity,* sec. ed. 1818.

Hall, Mr and Mrs S.C., *Ireland: its Character and Scenery,* 3 vol. London 1841.

Halliday Andrew, *A general view of the present state of lunatics and lunatic asylums in Great Britain and Ireland.* Edinburgh 1828.

Handlin Oscar, *Bostons immigrants 1790-1865; a study in*

acculturation. Massachusetts 1941.

Hancock W. Neilson, On the assimilation of the law in England, Scotland and Ireland as to the care of lunatics and their property in JSSISI viii, 1879-85.

Hancock W. Neilson ed., *Ancient Laws and Institutes of Ireland,* 6 vols. Dublin 1865-1901.

Harris Leslie, *Law and practice in lunacy in Ireland.* Dublin 1930.

Harty William, *Observations on an act for amending the law relating to private lunatic asylums in Ireland.* Dublin 1843.

Harty William, *Vindiciae medicae; an appeal to public opinion.* Dublin 1843.

Hodder Edwin, *The Life and Work of the Seventh Earl of Shaftesbury,* 3 vols. London 1886.

Howard John, *The State of the Prisons in England and Wales etc.* London 1784.

Howard John, *An Account of the Principal Lazarettos in Europe.* London 1789.

Jackson Thomas, *Remarks on Dr Jacob's pamphlet respecting the bye-laws for the district asylum in Ireland.* Armagh 1834.

Jones Kathleen, *Lunacy, Law and Conscience 1744-1845.* London 1955.

Jones Kathleen, *A History of the Mental Health Services.* London 1972.

John David, *Mental Handicap – an Introduction.* London 1976.

Joyce James, *Ulysses.* London 1937 ed.

Joyce P.W., *A Social History of Ancient Ireland,* 2 vol. London 1903.

Joyce P.W., *The Origin and History of Irish Names of Places,* 3 vol. Dublin 1895.

Kelly Tim, Ennis County Jail in *North Munster Antiquarian Journal* xvi (1973-4).

Kennedy Robert E. Jnr., *The Irish: Emigration, Marriage and Fertility.* California 1973.

Kennedy R.I., Physical Methods of Treatment in *Companion to Psychiatric Studies,* sec. ed.

Kenny Eyre E.C., *Short hints and observations on the arrangement and management of lunatic asylums.* Dublin 1848.

Kidd George G., *An appeal on behalf of the idiotic and imbecile children of Ireland, 1886.*

Kilkenny Archaeological Society, *Transactions* ii (1852-3).

Kingsley Charles, *His Letters and Memories of His Life* ed. his wife, 2 vols. London 1877.

Kirkpatrick T. Percy, *A note on the history of the care of the insane in Ireland up to the end of the nineteenth century.* Dublin 1931.

Lalor Joseph, On the use of education and training in the treatment of the insane in public lunatic asylums 1878 in JSSISI.

Latocnaye Marquis de, *Promenade d'un Francais dans l'Irlande 1796-7.* Dublin 1917.

The Legacy of Swift: a Bi-centenary Record of St Patrick's Hospital. Dublin 1948.

Lewin Walter ed., *Prose Writings of Swift.* London.

Letchworth William P., *The Insane in Foreign Countries.* New York 1889.

Litton Falkiner C., The History of St John of Jerusalem in Ireland in *Proceedings of the Royal Irish Academy* xxvi (1906).

Lloyd T.O., *Empire to Welfare State.* Oxford 1979.

Logan Patrick, *The Holy Wells of Ireland.* Buckinghamshire 1980.

Logan Patrick, Folk Medicine in the Cavan-Leitrim area, in *Ulster Folklife* ii, 1965.

Lonergan Eamonn, *St Luke's Hospital Clonmel 1884-1984.* 1984.

Lucas Charles, *The Theory and uses of Baths.* 1772.

Lyons J.B., Mercers Hospital 1734-1972 in *Journal of the Irish Medical Association* lxv (12). 1972.

MacDonagh Oliver, *Ireland; the Union and its Aftermath,* first ed. London 1968.

MacDonagh Oliver, *The Inspector General.* London 1981.

MacEoin Gearoid S., Gleann Bolcain agus Gleann na nGealt, *Béaloideas* xxx. 1962.

MacGill Patrick J., *The Parish of Killaghter.*

McKenna John, John Cicade, A Case for Treatment? in *Caritas* 46 (38).

Maloney Michael P. and Ward Michael P., *Mental Retardation and Modern Society.* Oxford 1970.

Maudsley Henry, *Body and Mind* rev. ed. 1873.

Mason William Shaw, *Parochial Survey of Ireland,* 2 vols. Dublin 1816.

McDowell R.B., *The Irish Administration 1801-1914.* London 1964.

McKeown Thomas, The concept of a balanced hospital community in *Lancet* i. 1958.

McNeill Charles, The Hospitallers at Kilmainham in *Journal of the Royal Society of Antiquaries* liv. 1924.

Meyer Kuno ed., *Cath Finntraga.* Oxford 1885.

Miller David W., *Church, State and Nation in Ireland 1898-1921.* Dublin 1973.

Moore J.N.P., *Swift's Philanthropy.* Dublin 1967.

Mora George, Historical and Theoretical trends in psychiatry in *Comprehensive Textbook of Psychiatry* 1967.

Morrin James, *Calendar of the Patent and Close Rolls of Chancery in Ireland from 18th to the 45th of Queen Elizabeth,* 2 vol. Dublin 1861.

Moylan Thomas King, Vagabonds and Sturdy Beggars in *Dublin Historical Record* i (3). 1938.

Mulcahy Michael, *Census of the Mentally Handicapped in the Republic of Ireland 1974.* Medico-Social Research Board.

Murphy Donal A. ed., *Tumbling Walls: the evolution of a community institution over 150 years.* Nenagh 1983.

New Catholic Encyclopedia, 17 vol. New York 1967.

Norman Connolly, *The family care of the insane.* London 1906.

Norman Connolly, *The domestic treatment of the insane.* Dublin 1896.

Norman Connolly, *Presidential address, fifty-third annual meeting of Medico-Psychological Association.* Lewes 1894.

Norman Connolly, *Family care of persons of unsound mind.*

Dublin 1903.

O'Brien George, *The Economic History of Ireland.* London 1921.

O'Brien Liam, The Magic Wisp: A history of the Mentally III in Ireland in *Bulletin of the Menninger Clinic* xxi (2). 1967.

O'Curry Eugene, *Manners and Customs of the Ancient Irish,* three vol. Dublin 1873.

O'Donoghue Edward G., *The Story of Bethlehem Hospital.* London 1914.

O'Donovan John trans., *Annals of Ireland — Three Fragments.* Dublin 1860.

O'Donovan John, *Ordnance Survey Letters (Donegal) 1835;* Kerry (1841).

O'Donovan John trans., *The Banquet of Dun na nGedh and the Battle of Magh Rath.* Dublin 1842.

O'Grady Standish ed. and trans., *Silva Gadelica — A Collection of Tales in Irish,* 2 vol. London 1892.

O'Hare Aileen and Dermot Walsh, *Irish Psychiatric Hospitals and Units Census 1981.* Dublin 1983.

O'Hare Aileen and Dermot Walsh, *Activities of Irish Psychiatric Hospitals and Units 1965-1982.*

O'Keefe J.G. trans., *Buile Suibhne (the frenzy of Suibhne) being the adventures of Suibhne Geilt,* Irish Texts Society xii. London 1913.

O'Muirgheasa Enri, The Holy Wells of Donegal in *Béaloideas* vi. 1936.

O'Rahilly T.F., Notes Mainly Etymological in *Eriú* xii. 1952.

Orrery John Earl of, *Remarks on the Life and Writings of Dr Jonathan Swift.* Dublin 1757.

O'Shea Brian and Falvey Jane, A History of St Brendan's Hospital Dublin in *Psychiatric Nursing.* Autumn 1984.

O'Tuathaigh Gearoid, *Ireland Before the Famine 1798-1848.* Dublin 1972.

Otway Caesar, *Sketches in Erris and Tyrawly.* London 1845.

Phelan Denis, *A Statistical Inquiry into the present state of the medical charities of Ireland.* Dublin 1835.

Pim Jonathan, On the necessity of state provision for the

education of the deaf, dumb, blind and imbecile in JSSISI (1868), pp. 26-41.

Plumer Charles ed., *Bethada Naem n-Eirinn; lives of Irish Saints,* 2 vols. Oxford 1922.

Prendergast F. Jarleth ed., Ancient History of the Kingdom of Kerry by Friar O'Sullivan in *Journal of Cork Historical and Archaelogical Society* sec. series vi. 1900.

Reid Thomas, *Travels in Ireland in 1822.* London 1823.

Reynolds Joseph, Glimpses of the Past in *Newsletter* (Mental Health Association of Ireland) ii (2).

Robins Joseph, The Irish Hospital in *Administration* viii (2), pp. 148-150.

Robins Joseph, *The Lost Children; a Study of Charity Children in Ireland 1700-1900.* Dublin 1980.

Robinson Henry, *Memories: Wise and Otherwise.* London 1924.

Rosen George, *Madness in Society.* London 1968.

Ross Chisholm, *Statistics of Insanity in New South Wales with reference to the Census of 1891 in Commitment Detention Care and Treatment of the Insane.*

Rossi Mario M. and Hone Joseph, *Swift.* 1978.

Rowland Peter, *Lloyd George,* London 1975.

Russell Jeffy Burton, *Witchcraft in the Middle Ages.* London 1972.

St Patrick's Hospital Dublin, Charter, bye-laws and will of founder. Dublin 1831.

Schrier Arnold, *Ireland and the American Emigration 1850-1900.* New York 1958.

Scull Andrew T., *Museums of Madness.* London 1979.

Scull Andrew T. ed., *Madhouses, Mad Doctors and Madmen.* London 1981.

Sheehan J. and de Barra E., *Ospideil na nEireann 1930-1955.*

Seymour St John D., *Irish Witchcraft and Demonology.* Dublin 1913.

Sigerson George, The Law and the Lunatic in JSSISI ix.

Skultans Vieda, *Madness and Morals: Ideas on Insanity in the Nineteenth Century.* London 1975.

Smith Charles, *The Ancient and Present State of the County of Kerry.* Dublin 1756.

Smith Roland M., The Advice to Diodin in *Eriú* xi. 1932.

Standing rules and regulations on the Royal Irish Constabulary 6th ed. Dublin 1911.

Stewart's Hospital, *Centenary Year Book.* Dublin 1969.

Stokes W.H. and Windisch E., *Coir Anmann,* Irsche Texte Leipzig, 1897.

Stokes W.H. trans., The Battle of Allen in *Revue Celtique* xxiv. 1903.

Swift Jonathan ed. Kathleen Williams, *A Tale of the Tub and other Satires.* London 1975.

Thernstrom Stephen, *Social Mobility in a Nineteenth Century City.* Harvard 1964.

Tucker George A., *Lunacy in Many Lands.* Sydney 1887.

Tuke Daniel Hack, *Chapters on the History of the Insane in the British Isles.* London 1882.

Tuke Harrington, On Warm and Cold Baths in the Treatment of Insansity in *Journal of Medical Science* iv (1858).

Valliant George E., *The Natural History of Alcholism.* London 1983.

Viney Michael, *Mental Illness.* Dublin 1963.

Walk Alexander, On the State of Lunacy 1859-1959 in *The Journal of Mental Science* cv (441). 1959.

Walsh Dermot, *The 1963 Irish Psychiatric Hospital Census.*

Wakeman W.F., *Three Days on the Shannon: From Limerick to Lough Key.* Dublin 1852.

Watson John, *The Gentleman's and Citizens Almanack 1752.* Dublin.

Weld Isaac, *Statistical Survey of the County of Roscommon.* Dublin 1832.

Welsford Enid, *The Fool – His Social and Literary History.* London 1935.   1935.

Wesley John, *Primitive Physic or an easy and natural Method of Curing most Diseases.* Twenty first ed. 1785.

Widdess J.D.H., *A Dublin School of Medicine and Surgery.* Edinburgh 1949.

Widdess J.D.H., *A History of the Royal College of Physicians of Ireland 1654-1963.* Edinburgh 1963.

Widdess J.D.H., *The Richmond, Whitworth and Hardwicke*

Hospitals, St. Laurence's Hospital Dublin 1772-1972. Dublin 1972.

Wilde Lady Jane Francesca, *Ancient Cures, Charms and Usanges of Ireland.* London 1890.

Wilde W.R., *The Closing Years of Dean Swift's Life.* Dublin 1849.

Wilde W.R., Some particulars respecting Swift and Stella with engravings of their crania etc. in *Dublin Quarterly Journal of Medical Science* iv. 1847.

Williams Harold, *Correspondence of Jonathan Swift.* 5 vol. London 1965.

Williamson Arthur, The Beginnings of State Care for the Mentally Ill in Ireland in *The Economic and Social Review* i (2). Dublin 1970.

Williamson Claude, Witchcraft in *The Irish Ecclesiastical Record,* fifth series xlii. 1933.

Wilson T.G., Swift and the Doctors in *Medical History* viii (3). 1964.

Wittke Carl, *The Irish in America.* Louisianna 1956.

Wood-Martin W.G., *Traces of the Elder Faiths of Ireland,* 2 vol. London 1902.

Wynter Andrew and Granville J. Mortimer, *The Borderlines of Insanity and other Papers.* London 1877.

Newspapers and Journals

Dublin Evening Mail
Dublin Journal of Medical Science
Dublin University Magazine
Freeman's Journal
Irish Independent
Irish Times
Journal of Mental Science
Limerick Chronicle
Nenagh Guardian
Nenagh News

Sligo Independent
Tuam Herald

Annual Reports of Public Institutions

Reports of district asylums:
Armagh 1828
Ballinasloe 1910
Belfast 1831, 1910
Cork 1828, 1910
Derry 1910
Enniscorthy 1902
Monaghan 1910
Mullingar 1902-3
Omagh 1902
Sligo 1910.

Annual Reports of Statutory Agencies

Deputy Keeper of the Public Records in Ireland 1869-1920.
Home Office (Northern Ireland) Services 1927-1938.
Inspectors for Ireland under the Inebriate Acts 1904-1916.
Inspectors of Lunatics in Ireland 1845-1922 (the last report
    was not published).
Inspectors of Lunacy, Northern Ireland 1924-1926.
Inspector of Mental Hospitals 1923-1961, 1977-1979.
Inspector-General of Prisons in Ireland 1815-1877.
Local Government Board for Ireland 1872-1921.

Parliamentary Papers and Government Publications

Pre-Union Irish Parliament
Report of committee to enquire into state of gaols. Irish
    House of Commons November 1729 (Pamphlet, National
    Library).
Report of committee on state and management of the fund
    of the workhouse of the City of Dublin. April 1758.
    Comms. jn. Ire. vi.
Report from the committee to whom the petition of the

governors of St Patrick's Hospital was referred. November 1763. Comms jn. Ire. vii.

Report from committee on petition of governors of St Patrick's. November 1767. Comms. jn. Ire. viii.

Report from committee on state of house of industry and its funds. May 1778. Comms. jn. Ire. ix.

Reports of committees on state of gaols prisons and bridewells. June 1782. Comms. jn. Ire. x; December 1783 Comms. jn. Ire. xi; May 1785 Comms. jn. Ire. xi.

Report of committee to enquire into the causes why the law respecting gaols and prisons had not been complied with etc. April 1787. Comms. jn. Ire. xii.

Report on the state of hospitals, infirmaries and public dispensaries. April 1788. Comms. jn. Ire. xii.

Report from committee appointed to examine the physicians who have attended His Majesty during his illness. February 1789. Comms. jn. Ire. xiii.

Petition of the acting governors of the house of industry. January 1793. Comms. jn. Ire. xvii.

A report on the prisons of Ireland for 1797 by the inspector general. March 1798. Comms. jn. Ire. xvii.

United Kingdom Parliament

Report of committee to consider the legislative provisions already existing for the support of the aged and infirm poor of Ireland etc. June 1804 H.C. 1803-4 (papers 61-150).

Report to lord lieutenant on certain charitable establishments in the City of Dublin etc. by John David Latouche, William Disney and George Penny. August 1808.

Report of committee to enquire into state prisons and other gaols in Ireland. May 1809 H.C. 1809 (265) vii.

Report from the committee on madhouses in England. July 1815 H.C. 1814-15 (296) iv.

Report from select committee on the lunatic poor Ireland. 1817 H.C. 1817 (430) viii.

Report of select committee on the state of gaols 1819 H.C. vii (579) 1819.

First report from select committee on the state of disease and condition of the labouring poor in Ireland. May 1819 H.C. 1819 (314) vii.

Report of commissioners appointed by the lord-lieutenant to inspect the house of industry etc. May 1820 H.C. 1820 (84) viii.

House of Industry Dublin: correspondence. May 1821 H.C. 1821 (587) xx.

An account of lunatics and idiots at present confined and maintained . . . in Ireland. H.C. 1826 (289) xxiii.

Correspondence and communications between the Home Office and the Irish government, 1827, on the subject of private lunatic asylums. H.C. 1828 (234) xxii.

Report of select committee on Irish miscellaneous estimates. June 1829 H.C. 1829 (342) iv.

Report of select committee on the state of the poor in Ireland. 1830 H.C. 1830 (667) vii.

Charitable institutions, Dublin; reports of commissioners appointed by lord-lieutenant. February 1830 H.C. 1830 (7) xxvi.

Report from select committee on county cess (Ireland) 1836 H.C. 1836 (527) xii.

Three reports of commissioners for enquiry into the conditions of the poorer classes in Ireland. First H.C. 1835 (369) xxxii pts. 1 and 2; second 1837 (68) xxxi; third 1836 (43) xxx.

Poor Laws-Ireland; three reports by George Nicholls etc. H.C. 1837 (69) li; 1837 (104) xxxviii; 1837 (126) xxxviii.

Tables of the revenue, population, commerce etc. of the United Kingdom and its dependencies, part iv. 1836. H.C. 1837-8 (280) xlvii.

Report select committee, House of Lords, on the state of the lunatic poor in Ireland 1843. H.C. 1843 (625) x.

Lunatic asylums (Ireland): Returns for year ending 31-3-1844. H.C. 1844 (472) xliii.

Lunatic poor (Ireland). Correspondence between the Irish government and the managers of district lunatic asylums 1844. H.C. 1844 (233) xliii.

Correspondence between the Irish government and grand juries on the subject of additional accommodation for pauper lunatics 1844 H.C. 1844 (603) xliii.

Select committee lunatic asylums (Ireland) (advances) bill; minutes of evidence. May 1855 H.C. 1854-5 (262) viii.

District lunatic asylums (Ireland): report etc. of commission into the erection of district lunatic asylums in Ireland. December 1855 H.C. 1856 (9) liii.

Report and minutes of evidence of commissioners of enquiry into the state of lunatic asylums etc. in Ireland 1858. H.C. 1857-8 (10) xxvii.

Observations on the report of the commissioners . . . J. Nugent, Inspector of lunatic asylums. October 1858 H.C. 1859 (147 sess. 1) xxii.

Lunatic asylums (Ireland) commission: communication of Dr D.J. Corrigan assigning his reasons for dissenting etc. February 1859 H.C. 1859 (95) xxii.

Lunacy (Ireland) number, names and qualifications of the commissioners of control in lunacy in Ireland July 1869 H.C. 1868-9 (389) li.

Lunatic Asylums (Cork etc): return of places in which Turkish baths have been created etc. July 1870 H.C. 1870 (372) lvii.

Report and minutes of evidence select committee on lunacy law. April 1877 H.C. 1878 (113) xvi.

Report and minutes of evidence poor law union and lunacy inquiry (Ireland) 1879 H.C. 1878-9 (2239) xxxi.

Union Workhouses (Ireland) (sick persons) H.C. 1881 (443) lxxix.

First and second reports of the commission appointed by the lord-lieutenant of Ireland on lunacy administration (Ireland) 1891 H.C. 1890-91 (6434) xxxvi.

Report of select committee on Belfast Corporation (lunatic asylums etc.) bill 1892 H.C. 1892 (228) xi.

Memorandum of Lord Ashbourne, lord chancellor of Ireland on the reports of the committee on lunacy administration appointed by the lord-lieutenant April 1892. HMSO Dublin 1892.

Report and minutes of evidence of the vice-regal commission on poor law reform in Ireland. 1906 H.C. 1906 (3202) li; 1906 (3204) lii.

Report of royal commission on the care and control of the feeble minded 1908 H.C. 1908 (4202) xxxix.

Report from select committee on asylum officers superannuation bill 1909 H.C. 1909 (257) vi.

Report of royal commission on the poor law and relief of distress – report on Ireland H.C. 1909 (4630) xxxviii. Minutes of evidence H.C. 1910 (5070) 1.

A hospital plan for England and Wales. HMSO 1962.

Northern Ireland

Reports of select committee on health services in Northern Ireland. Belfast HMSO 1944.

Report of mental health services committee on mental deficiency in Northern Ireland. Belfast HMSO 1946.

The future mental health service of Northern Ireland. Belfast HMSO 1948.

Report of a sub-committee of the standing medical advisory committee for Northern Ireland on geriatric and psychiatric services for the elderly. Belfast HMSO 1970.

Consultative document on services for the mentally handicapped. Department of Health and Social Services. Belfast 1976.

Services for the mentally handicapped in Northern Ireland; policy and objectives. July 1978 Belfast HMSO.

Psychiatric hospitals in Northern Ireland: a survey. March 1979 Department of Health and Social Services. Belfast.

Northern Ireland: review committee on mental health legislation. October 1981. Belfast HMSO.

Republic of Ireland

Report of the commission on the relief of the sick and destitute poor including the insane poor 1927.

Reconstruction and improvement of county homes 1952 (pr. 756).

The problem of the mentally handicapped 1960 (pr. 5456).

Report of commission of inquiry on mental handicap 1965 (pr. 8234).

The health services and their future development: a white paper 1966 (pr. 8653).

Report of commission of inquiry on mental illness 1966 (pr. 9181).

Outline of the future hospital system: report of the consultative council on the general hospital services 1967 (pr. 154).

Psychiatric nursing services of health boards – report of working party 1973 (pr. 3043).

Interdepartmental committee on mentally ill and maladjusted persons. First interim report: Assessment services for the courts in respect of juveniles 1974 (pr. 4688); Second interim report: The provision of treatment for juvenile offenders and potential juvenile offenders 1974 (pr. 4689); Third interim report: Treatment and care of persons suffering from mental disorder who appear before the courts on criminal charges 1978 (pr. 8275).

Training and employing the handicapped: report of a working party established by the Minister for Health 1975 (pr. 4302).

Services for the mentally handicapped: report of a working party 1980 (pr. 8489).

Statistical information relevant to the health services. Department of Health 1984.

Towards a full life: green paper on services for disabled people 1984 (pr. 2264).

The psychiatric services: planning for the future 1985 (pr. 3001).

Parliamentary Debates
Dail Eireann Debates 1922-1980.

Hansard Parliamentary Debates.

Journals of Irish House of Commons 1613-1800. Dublin 1796-1980.

Journals of Irish House of Lords 1634-1800. Dublin 1799-1800.

The Parliamentary Register or history of the proceedings and debates of the House of Commons of Ireland 1781-97, 17 vols. Dublin 1782-1801.

List of statutes in whole or in part regulating or influencing provisions for mentally ill persons (including inebriates) in the Republic of Ireland and Northern Ireland.

Pre-Union Irish Parliament
1634-5   10 and 11 Car. 1. c.4.
1634-5   10 and 11 Car. 1. c. 16.
1703   2 Anne c. 19.
1729   3 Geo. 2. c. 17.
1763   3 Geo. 3. c. 5.
1763   3 Geo. 3. c. 28.
1765   5 and 6 Geo. 3. c. 10.
1772   11 and 12 Geo. 3. c. 30.
1786   26 Geo. 3. c. 27.
1787   27 Geo. 3. c. 39.

United Kingdom Parliament
1324   17 Edw. 2. c. 9.
1639   Ch. 1. c. 53.
1774   14 Geo. 3. c. 7.
1800   39 and 40 Geo. 3. c. 94.
1805   45 Geo. 3. c. 111.
1806   46 Geo. 3. c. 95.
1808   48 Geo. 3. c. 96.
1815   55 Geo. 3. c. 107.
1817   57 Geo. 3. c. 106.
1818   58 Geo. 3. c. 47.
1820   1 Geo. 4. c. 98.
1821   1 and 2 Geo. 4. c. 33.
1822   3 Geo. 4. c. 64.
1825   6 Geo. 4. c. 53.
1825   6 Geo. 4. c. 54.
1826   7 Geo. 4. c. 14.
1826   7 Geo. 4. c. 74.

1829	10 Geo. 4. c. 34.
1830	11 Geo. 4. c. 22.
1831	1 Will. 4. c. 13.
1831	1 Will. 4. c. 65.
1835	5 and 6 Will. 4. c. 17.
1836	6 and 7 Will. 4. c. 116.
1837	1 and 2 Vic. c. 27.
1842	5 and 6 Vic. c. 123.
1843	6 and 7 Vic. c. 92.
1845	8 and 9 Vic. c. 107.
1846	9 and 10 Vic. c. 79.
1846	9 and 10 Vic. c. 115.
1847	10 Vic. c. 31.
1849	12 and 13 Vic. c. 56.
1851	14 and 15 Vic. c. 45.
1851	14 and 15 Vic. c. 68.
1852	15 and 16 Vic. c. 48.
1855	18 and 19 Vic. c. 76.
1855	18 and 19 Vic. c. 109.
1856	19 and 20 Vic. c. 99.
1861	24 and 25 Vic. c. 57.
1867	30 and 31 Vic. c. 118.
1868	31 and 32 Vic. c. 97.
1871	34 Vic. c. 22.
1874	37 and 38 Vic. c. 74.
1875	38 and 39 Vic. c. 67.
1877	40 and 41 Vic. c. 27.
1878	41 and 42 Vic. c. 60.
1879	42 and 43 Vic. c. 19.
1880	43 and 44 Vic. c. 39.
1883	46 and 47 Vic. c. 38.
1883	46 and 47 Vic. c. 42.
1884	47 and 48 Vic. c. 64.
1887	50 and 51 Vic. c. 16.
1887	50 and 51 Vic. c. 67.
1888	51 and 52 Vic. c. 19.
1890	53 Vic. c. 5.
1890	53 and 54 Vic. c. 31.

1892	55 and 56 Vic. c. 231.
1893	56 and 57 Vic. c. 65.
1897	60 Vic. c. 37.
1898	61 and 62 Vic. c. 37.
1898	61 and 62 Vic. c. 60.
1899	62 and 63 Vic. c. 32.
1901	1 Edw. 7. c. 17.
1909	9 Edw. 7. c. 48.
1913	3 and 4 Geo. 5. c. 28.
1914	4 and 5 Geo. 5. c. 58.
1919	9 and 10 Geo. 5. c. 96.
1920	10 and 11 Geo. 5. c. 67.
1927	17 and 18 Geo. 5. c. 23.
1930	20 and 21 Geo. 5. c. 23.
1946	9 and 10 Geo. 6. c. 81.
1947	10 and 11 Geo. 6. c. 37.
1959	7 and 8 Eliz. 2. c. 72.
1960	8 and 9 Eliz. 2. c. 61.
1978	26 and 27 Eliz. 2. c.28.
1978	26 and 27 Eliz. 2. c. 52.

Northern Ireland Parliament

Mental Health Act (N.I.) 1932 (22 and 23 Geo. 5. c. 15)
Health Services Act (N.I.) 1948 (c.3.)
Mental Health Act (N.I.) 1948 (c. 17.)
Mental Health Act (N.I.) 1961 (c. 15.)
Health Services (Amendment) Act (N.I.) 1963 (c. 20.)

Irish Parliament

Adaptation of Enactments Act 1922 (No. 2)
Local Government (Temporary Provisions) Act 1923 (No. 2)
Ministers and Secretaries Act 1924 (No. 16)
Local Government Act 1925 (No. 5)
Public Charitable Hospitals (Amendment) (No. 2) Act 1931
   (No. 49)
Public Charitable Hospitals (Amendment) (No. 3) Act1931
   (No. 51)
Public Hospitals Act 1933 (No. 18)

Public Hospitals (Amendment) Act 1938 (No. 21)

Hospitals Act 1939 (No. 4)

Public Hospitals (Amendment) (No. 2) Act 1939 (No. 29)

Public Hospitals (Amendment) Act 1940 (No. 9)

Mental Treatment Act 1945 (No. 19)

Ministers and Secretaries (Amendment) Act 1946 (No. 3)

Nurses Act 1950 (No. 27)

Health Act 1953 (No. 26)

Mental Treatment Act 1953 (No. 35)

Health and Mental Treatment Act 1957 (No. 16)

Health and Mental Treatment (Amendment) Act 1958 (No. 37)

Health Authorities Act 1960 (No. 9)

Criminal Justice Act 1960 (No. 27)

Mental Treatment (Detention in Approved Institutions) Act 1961 (No. 4)

Mental Treatment Act 1961 (No. 7)

Nurses Act 1961 (No. 18)

Health Act 1970 (No. 1)

Health (Mental Services) Act 1981 (No. 17)

References

Chapter 1.

1. Connellan trans. *Four Masters*, p. 1.
2. Rosen, *Madness in Society*, pp. 28, 77, 90.
3. *Coir Anmann*, p. 367.
4. Plummer trans. *Bethada Naem n Erenn* ii, p. 285; Cambrensis, *Historical Works*, pp. 97, 106.
5. Meyer trans. *Cath Finntraga*, pp. 17, 18.
6. Wood Martin, *Traces of the Elder Faiths* i, p. 352.
7. O'Donovan trans. *Annals of Ireland: Three Fragments*, p. 41; Stokes trans. *The Battle of Allen*, p. 55.
8. Camden, *Britannia*, p. 798.
9. O'Donovan trans. *The Banquet of Dun na nGedh and the Battle of Magh Rath*, pp. 231-237; O'Keefe trans. *Buile Suibhne*.
10. Smith, The advice to Doidin in *Eriú* xi, pp. 65-85.
11. O'Rahilly, Notes, Mainly Etymological in *Eriú* xiii, pp. 149-150.
12. Binchy, Bretha Crólige in *Eriú* xii, pp. 12, 13, 59.
13. Chadwick, Geilt in *Scottish Gaelic Studies* v, pt. 2, pp. 107-125.
14. *Transactions Kilkenny Arch. Soc.* ii, p. 5; Folklore Archives 1223 (59); Wood Martin *op. cit.* i, pp. 355-356.
15. Eachard, *An Exact Description of Ireland*, p. 21.
16. Folklore Archives 744 (567); 433 (371).
17. Mac Eoin, Gleann Bolcain agus Gleann na nGealt in *Béaloideas* xxx, pp. 105-120.
18. Folklore Archives 692 (171-177); 782 (363); 1564 (161); O'Donovan, *Ordnance Survey Letters (Kerry)*, pars. 122-125; Joyce, *Irish Names of Places* i, pp. 172-173.
19. Prendergast ed, Ancient History of the Kingdom of Kerry in *Jn. Cork Hist. Arch. Soc.* vi (second series), p. 103.
20. O'Donovan *op. cit.*, pp. 122-125.
21. Folklore Archives 1066 (83-85); 858 (432-436); 47 (241).
22. Folklore Archives 1564 (161); 1006 (399-410); Prendergast

op. cit., p. 103 fn.; Tuke, *History of Insane in the British Isles*, p. 23.

23. O'Muirgheasa, The Holy Wells of Donegal in *Béaloideas* vi, p. 157; O'Donovan, *Ordnance Survey Letters (Donegal)*, pars. 171-172.

24. Mason, *Parochial Survey of Ireland* ii, p. 181; Folk-lore Archives 1358 (143).

25. McGill, *The Parish of Killaghter*, p. 5.

26. Logan Folk-medicine in the Cavan-Leitrim area, *Ulster Folklife* ii, 1965.

27. Logan, *The Holy Wells of Ireland*, p. 73.

28. Wakeman, *Three Days on the Shannon*, pp. 46-47.

Chapter 2

1. Senchus Mor i, pp. 50, 53, 157, 163, 201, 203; iii, pp. 11, 12, 157.

2. *ibid* i, pp. 125, 137, 139.

3. *ibid* ii, p. 407; iii, pp. 199-201; v, p. 493.

4. Welsford, *The Fool: His Social and Literary History*.

5. *ibid*, p. 55.

6. O'Grady trans. *Silva Gadelica* ii, pp. 116-117.

7. Welsford, op. cit. pp. 113-182.

8. Tuke, *Chapters in the History of the Insane in the British Isles*, pp. 8-9.

9. Gwynn and Hadcock, *Medieval Religious Houses in Ireland*.

10. Archdall, *Monasticon Hibernicum*, p. 647.

11. Henry Ellis ed., *Original Letters Illustrative of English History* third series iv, p. 61.

12. Russell, *Witchcraft in the Middle Ages*, pp. 60, 301n.

13. Cohn, *Europe's Inner Demons*, pp. 21-23, 121-122.

14. Williamson, Witchcraft in *Irish Ecclesiastical Record* 5th series xlii, pp. 262-272.

15. Rosen *op. cit.*, pp. 238-241.

16. *Dublin University Magazine* lxvi, pp. 473-476; Russell *op. cit.*, p. 189.

17. Cohn *op. cit.*, p. 202.

18. Seymour, *Irish Witchcraft and Demonology*, pp. 59-61.

19. *ibid*, pp. 105-131.

20. Hall, *Ireland: Its Scenery and Character* iii, p. 125.

21. Burdett *op. cit.* i, p. 51; 9 Geo. 2 c, 5; 10 Geo. 4 c, 34, s. i.

22. *Journ. Roy. Soc. Antiq. Ire.* xxv, p. 84.

23. *Journ. Cork Hist. Arch. Soc.* viii sec. series, p. 122.

Chapter 3

1. Burton, *The Anatomy of Melancholy* 1806 ed. i, p. xvii.
2. *ibid*, p. 85.
3. Davies, *Why are People so Cruel?*; Burdett, *Hospitals and Asylums of the World* i, p. 62.
4. *Commons jn. Ire.* XIII, app. xi.
5. Logan, *The Holy Wells of Ireland*, p. 74.
6. Harrington Tuke, *On Warm and Cold Baths in the Treatment of Insanity*.
7. John Wesley, *Primitive Physic, or an Easy and Natural Method of Curing Most Diseases,* twenty-first ed. p. 77.
8. Lucas, *The Therapy and Uses of Baths*.
9. *Ancient Cures Charms and Usages of Ireland*, p. 33.
10. Morrin, *Calendar of the Patent and Close Rolls* ii, p. 163-164; *Seventh Rep. deputy keeper public records Ire.* app. x, 431 (514).
11. 10 and 11 Car. 1, c. 4.
12. 10 and 11 Car. 1, c. 16.
13. *Cal. Anc. Rec. Dub.* v 321; vi 257; *Census of Ireland 1851: Report on Status of Disease*, p. 62.
14. *Commons jn. Ire.* v, 708-722; *Rep. comm. enq. state of gaols* 1729, Commons jn. Ire. iii (pt 2), app. ccclxxxvi.
15. Elrington Ball, *The Correspondence of Dean Swift* iv, pp. 343-348.
16. *Rep. comm. management fund workhouse* 1758 Commons jn. Ire. vi, pp. xcvi-c.
17. 3 Geo. 3, c. 5, Ir stat.; 3 Geo. 3, c. 28, Ir stat.
18. *Parliamentary Register* iii, pp. 89-90, 118; Howard, *Works* ii, pp. 79-80; Edward Foster, *A letter to Sydenham Singleton Chairman of Committee to enquire into State of Lunatics etc 1777*.
19. Rep. comm state public prisons Dublin December 1783, *Commons jn. Ire.* xi, p. cxxxi; *Rep. comms. public prisons* May 1785 Comms jn. Ire. xi, pp. ccccxiii-ccccxv; McDonagh, *The Inspector-General*, pp. 56-83.
20. *Parl. Register* vii, p. 429.
21. 26 Geo. 3, c. 27, Ir. stat.; Fitzpatrick, *An Essay on Gaol Abuses etc*.
22. Geo. 3, c. 39.
23. McDonagh *op. cit.*, pp. 110, 118, 140-168.
24. *ibid*, p. 143.
25. O.P. 267/6, Trevor to James Trail 6/4/1808.
26. *Hansard* ii, pars. 1131-1132.
27. *Rep. comm. pris. Ire. 1809*, pp. 13-20, 70. H.C. 1809 (265).
28. *Report sel. comm. state of gaols* 1819, p. 206. H.C. 1819 (579) vii.
29. *Report insp. gen. prisons Ire.* 1823, pp. 8, 46, H.C. 1923 (342) x.
30. Fry and Gurney, *Report to Marquess Wellesly*.
31. Weld, *Statistical Survey of*

Roscommon, p. 423.

32. 3 Geo. 4, c. 64, ss. 13, 14; McDowell, *The Irish Administration*, pp. 48, 151.

33. 11 and 12 Geo. 3, c. 30, Ir. stat.

34. *Report comm. management H. of I.* November 1819, pp. 3-4. H.C. 1800 (84) viii.

35. *Rep. comm. state of H. of I. May 1778* Comms jn. Ire. ix, pp. dclxxiv-dclxxxiv.; *Rep. char. estab. Dublin* 1809, pp. 27-30; *Rep. sel. comm. lunatic poor Ire.* H.C. 1817 (430) viii, p. 24.

36. *Report* 1817, p. 14; *Hansard* iv, p. 66; O.P. 407 (3) 1814.

37. *Report 1817*, pp. 12-14; Reg. papers 407 (3) 1814; Carr, *The Stranger in Ireland*, p. 323.

38. *Promenade d'un Francais en Irlande*, pp. 63-64.

39. *Report comm. on madhouses England*, pp. 4, 5, 24 H.C. iv (296) 1814-5.

40. *Hansard* xxxv, par. 882.

41. Croker, *Researches in the South of Ireland*, pp. 34-35.

42. *Report sel. comm. poor Ire.* 1830 q 5707. H.C. 1830 (667) vii.

43. Anon, *Five Letters on the Poor of Ireland* 1816, pamph.

44. *Report* 1817, pp. 23-23; Fitzgerald and McGregor, *History of Limerick* i, p. 309.

45. Wilde, *Ancient Cures Charms and Usages of Ireland*, pp. 34-37.

46. 27 Geo. 3, c. 39, Ir. stat.

47. *Hansard* xxxv, par. 881.

48. *Report char. estab. Dublin 1809*, p. 43.

49. O.P. 409/2 1814.

50. *Report comm. madhouses England 1815*, pp. 4, 5, 181.

51. *ibid*, p. 24.

52. *Report 1817*, pp. 22, 23.

53. *Hansard* xxxv, par. 881.

Chapter 4

1. Lewin, *Prose Writings of Swift*, p. ix.

2. Williams ed. *A Tale of a Tub and other Satires*.

3. O'Donoghue, *The Story of Bethlehem Hospital*, pp. 249-251.

4. Ball, *The Correspondence of Jonathan Swift* i, p. 383; ii, p. 54 fn.; Williams, *The Correspondence of Jonathan Swift* ii, p. 425.

5. Davis ed. *Swift – Poetical Works*, pp. 601-608.

6. *Cal. Anc. Rec. Dub.* vi, p. 214.

7. 2 Anne c. 19, Ir. stat.

8. Ball op. cit. iv, pp. 343-348.

9. Fownes, *Methods proposed for regulating the poor etc.*

10. Ball. op. cit. pp. 343-348.

11. Robins, *The Lost Children*, p. 21.

12. Davis *op. cit.*, p. 513.

13. Williams, *Correspondence* v, p. 65.

14. Wilde, *Some particulars respecting Swift and Stella etc.* p. 28.
15. Robins, The Irish Hospital in *Administration* vii, (2). pp. 148-150.
16. *Wilde, op. cit.* p. 29; Wilde, *The Closing Years of Dean Swift's Life,* p. 82.
17. Ball. op. cit. vi, p. 48.
18. Craig in *The Legacy of Swift,* pp. 7-8.
19. Ball. op. cit. vi, pp. 85-88.
20. Gwynn, *The Life and Friendships of Dean Swift,* p. 306.
21. Wilson, Swift and the Doctors in *Medical History* viii (3) p. 202.
22. Orrery, *Remarks on the Life and Writings of Dr. Jonathan Swift,* p. 264.
23. Banks, The Writ *"de lunatico inquirendo"* in the case of Jonathan Swift etc. in *Dublin Quar. Jour. Med. Sc.* xxxi, pp. 83-90.
24. Joyce, *Ulysses* (London 1937 ed.), p. 36.
25. Orrery *op. cit.,* p. 266. St. Patrick's Hospital, Dublin, Charter.
26. Board Minutes 10/3/1746; 11/12/1747; 18/4/1749; 30/6/1749; 21/1/1751; 14/9/1757, 1/11/1763.
27. Board Minutes 10/3/1746; 30/6/1749; 2/2/1750; 1/11/1763.
28. *Commons jn. Ire.* vi, p. 234 and app. ccxxvii; *Commons jn. Ire.* vii, app. clxix; Board minutes 8/11/1800.
29. *The Legacy of Swift* appendix; Board minutes 29/7/1757.
30. Board minutes 12/8/1757.
31. Board minutes 23/12/1758; 7/5/1759; 16/7/1783; 8/11/1800.
32. Board minutes 23/1/1775.
33. *Comms. condition poor Ire.* First rep. app B, pp. 418-426, H.C. xxxii (pt. 2) 1835; *Third rep.* app. C, pt. 2, p. 67, H.C. xxx 1836.
34. *ibid third report,* p. 68.
35. *Report H.L. lunatic poor Ire.* 1843, qq 444-449; *Hospital Charter and Bye-Laws,* pp. 29-34.
36. *The Legacy of Swift,* p. 15.
37. *First rep. comms. condition poor Ire.* app. B, pp. 418-420.

Chapter 5

1. Tuke, *Chapters in the History of the Insane in the British Isles,* pp. 112-132.
2. Foucault, *Discipline and Punish,* pp. 8-20.
3. Tuke *op. cit.* 136-137.
4. Society of Friends papers PB 20 (107, 107a, 108, 109a); *Report sel. comm. H.L. lunatic poor Ire 1843,* qq 604-608 H.C. 1843 (625), x.
5. *Correspondence between Home Office and Irish Government 1827* app. 10 H.C. 1828 (234), xxiii.
6. *Report sel. comm. lunatic*

poor *Ireland* 1817, p. 12
H.C. 1817 (430), viii.

7. Hallaran, *Practical Observations on the Causes and Cure of Insanity* 1810 ed.

8. *Correspondence . . . 1827*, pp. 17-21.

9. Cummins, *Some Chapters of Cork Medical History*, pp. 27-32; *Fifth rep. ILI*, p. 13.

10. *Correspondence . . . 1827*, app. 10.

11. *Report sel. comm. aged and infirm poor Ireland etc. 1804* H.C. 1803-4 (109), iv.

12. *Hansard* iv, pars. 66, 206-208.

13. 46 Geo. iii, c. 95.

14. *Dictionary of National Biography* xxiv, pp. 358-359.

15. 15 Geo. iii, c. 9.

16. 48 Geo. iii, c. 96; Tuke *op. cit.* p. 165.

17. *A report upon certain charitable estabs etc.* 1809, pp. 41, 43.

18. *Report sel. comm. lunatic poor Ire.* 1843, pp. i-iii H.C. 1843 (625), x.

19. Robins *op. cit.*, pp. 10-59.

20. 55 Geo iii, c. 107.

21. O.P. 409(2), 1814.

22. Report to the governors July 1813 in *Newsletter of Mental Health Assn. of Ireland* ii, (2).

23. O.P. 409(2), 1814.

24. O.P. 407(3), 1814.

25. *Report lunatic poor* 1817, pp. 8-9; *Report commissioners on management H. of I May* 1820, p. 5 H.C. 1820 (84), viii.

26. Tuke, *op. cit.*, pp. 401-402; *Report insp. lun. Ire.*

1843, p. 5.

27. *Report sel. comm. madhouses England* July 1815, pp. 4-5 H.C. 1814-15 (296), iv.

28. *Hansard* xxxv (1817), par. 881.

29. *Report lunatic poor 1817.*

30. Halliday, *A general view of the present state of lunatics etc.*, p. 35; 57 Geo. iii, c. 106.

31. 1 Geo iv, c. 98.

32. 1 & 2 Geo iv, c. 33; 6 Geo iv, c. 54; 7 Geo iv, c. 14; 7 Geo iv, c. 74; 11 Geo iv, c. 22.

33. McDowell, *The Irish Administration 1802-1914*, p. 173.

34. O.P. 552(2) 1818; 59/47 (20) 1820.

35. *Report sel. comm. poor Ire.* 1830, pp. 28-29 H.C. 1830 (667), vii; 11 Geo iv, c. 22; 1 Will iv, c. 13.

36. *Summary reports sel. comm. poor Ire.* July 1830, p. 55 H.C. 1830 (667), vii.

37. Robins *op. cit.*, chapters 2 and 3.

38. Robins, The Irish Hospitals in *Administration* viii (2), pp. 146-165.

39. *ibid.*

40. 5 and 6 Geo. 3, c. 10.

41. Howard, *An Account of the Principal Lazarettos in Europe*, pp. 78-100.

42. *Poor enquiry (Ireland): first rep.* app. B, pp. 10-25.

43. Phelan, *A statistical enquiry etc.* app. ix.

44. 45 Geo. 3, c. 111; 58 Geo. 3, c. 47.

45. *Rep. sel. comm. disease labouring poor Ire. 1819* app. 2.
46. Phelan, *op. cit.* p. 56.
47. Widdess, *A History of the Royal College of Physicians of Ireland 1654-1963*; Widdess, *A Dublin School of Medicine and Surgery*.
48. 46 Geo. 3, c. 95.
49. *Rep. sel. comm. Irish misc. est. 1829*, pp. 13, 121.

50. Phelan, *op. cit.* pp. 37, 38.
51. MacDonagh, *Ireland*, p. 27.
52. *ibid*, pp. 7-8.
53. Phelan, *op. cit.* p. 262.
54. *Correspondence . . . 1827*, Spring Rice to William Lamb 20 July 1827.
55. *Dictionary of National Biography* xviii, pp. 835-837.
56. Monteagle papers MSS 548.
57. *ibid*, MSS 605.

Chapter 6

1. *Tables of the revenue, population, commerce etc. of the United Kingdom etc.* part vi 1836, tables 141, 142 H.C. 1837-8 (280), xlvii.
2. *Rep. sel. comm. 1843*, p. iv; qq 427-430.
3. *ibid*, pp. xiv-xxv.
4. *Rep. insp. general* 1844, p. 5.
5. Otway Caesar, *Sketches in Erris and Tyrawly*, p. 30.
6. *Corresp. between Irish gov. and grand juries* 1844 H.C. 1844 (603), xliii.
7. *First rep. ILI*, pp. 6-8; *sixth rep.*, pp. 3-7.
8. *Tenth rep. ILI*, pp. 3-4; Lonergan, *St Luke's Hospital Clonmel 1834-1984*, pp. 31-32.
9. *Rep. poor law and lun. enq. (Ire) 1879*, pp. lxxxvi-lxxvii H.C. 1878-9 (2239), xxxi; *Fifty-fourth rep. ILI*, p. xiv and supp. p. vii.
10. *Report comm enq. 1858* pt. 1, pp. 12-13.

11. Larcom papers MS 7775 Report to lords comms of the treasury . . . December 1855.
12. *ibid*.
13. *Mins. evid. sel. comm. lun. asy. Ire. advances Bill* 1855 qq 68-80 H.C. 1854-5 (262), viii.
14. *Rep. comms. enq.* 1858 pt. 2, q. 68.
15. *Mins. evid. sel. comm.* 1855 qq 13, 14.
16. Larcom pap. report December 1855.
17. Tuke *op. cit.*, pp. 147-174; *Census of Ireland* pt. 3, p. 65.
18. O.P. 407/2 (1814).
19. *ibid*; 407/6 (1814).
20. *Rep. insp. gen. prisons* 1823, pp. 25-30.
21. Hall, *Ireland; Its Scenery and Character* ii, p. 345.
22. 7 Geo 4, c. 74, 55, 61; 5 & 6 Vic., c. 123.
23. *Rep. insp. gen. pris. on asylums* 1843, sch. H.
24. *Twelfth rep ILI*, app. G.

25. Williamson in *The Economic and Social Review* i (2), p. 285.
26. *Fifty-fourth rep ILI*, p. xlviii.
27. *Fifth rep*, pp. 14-15; *sixth rep.*, p. 18; *eighth rep.*, p. 24; *rep. comms. enq.* 1858, pt. 2, qq 951, 969.
28. *ibid*, pt. 1, pp.32-36.
29. *Eighteenth rep. ILI*, p. 35.
30. *ibid.*
31. Tucker, *Lunacy in Many Lands*, p. 1277.
32. *Mins evid. sel. comm. lun. law* 1877, qq 2698-2749.
33. Burdett *op. cit.* i, p. 247.
34. *Observations on an Act for Amending the Law relating to Private Lunatic Asylums in Ireland 1843.*
35. Harty, *Vindiciae Medicae; an appeal to public opinion.*
36. Corbett in *Commitment, Detention and care of the Insane* (report of International Congress, Chicago 1893), pp. 44-48.
37. *ibid.*
38. *Mental Treatment Act* 1945.

Chapter 7

1. *Third rep. comms. poor Ire.*, p. 26 H.C. 1836 (43), xxx.
2. *Poor laws – Ireland; report by George Nicholls*, p. 30 H.C. 1837 (69), li.
3. *Rep. lun.poor* 1843, app. M.
4. *Provisional Government (Transfer of Functions) Order* 1922; *Adaptation of Enactments Act 1922; Ministers and Secretarys Act 1924.*
5. Larcom papers ms. 7775.
6. 18 & 19 Vic c. 109, s.5: *Tenth rep. ILI*, app. F.
7. *First & second reps. comm. lun. admin.* 1890-91, pp. 5-6.
8. *ibid*, pp. 3-6.
9. Papers Insp. Lun. memorandum, Lord Ashbourne to Earl of Zetland 25/6/1892.
10. 61 & 62 Vic., c. 37, s. 9.
11. 1 & 2 Geo. iv, c. 33, s. 5; *Rep. insp gen. pris. on asy.* 1843, app. 3.
12. 8 & 9 Vic., c. 107, ss. 23, 24.
13. Finnane *op. cit.*, p. 42.
14. *Rep. comms. enq. lunatic asylum Ire. 1858 pt 2,* qq 1262-1266; *Gen. rules and regs. management asy. Ire.* 1890, pp. 15-16.
15. O.P. 1833 (633).
16. *Rep. insp. gen. pris. asy.* 1843.
17. Jackson, *Remarks on Dr. Jacobs Pamphlet respecting the Bye-laws for the District Asylums in Ireland.*
18. *Lunatic (Poor) Ireland; correspondence ... 1844,* p. 3 H.C. 1844 (233), xliii; *Rep. lunatic poor Irel. 1843* qq 34-38.
19. Williamson *op. cit*, pp. 287-288.
20. *Rep. ins. gen. prisons 1843,* app. 3.
21. *Third rep. ILI 1848,* p. 4:

sixth rep. ILI 1853, p. 10;
ninth rep. ILI 1859, p. 13;
tenth rep. ILI 1861, app.
B. 20.
22. Reg. papers 1852 G2679.
23. *Rep. comms. enq. asylums
Ire.* 1858 pt. 2 qq 262,
5737,6242; Finnane *op. cit.*,
p. 64.
24. Mayo papers M.S. 11208
Letter from Dr. David Jacob
13-7-1867.
25. *Rep. 1858*, pt 2 qq 1750-
1760.
26. *ibid* qq 7220-7257.
27. *Journ. Ment. Sc.* vii (1861),
pp. 275-286.
28. *Rep. 1858* qq 327-330.
29. *Rep. 1858* pt. 1, p. 9.
30. *Lunatic asylums (Ire.)
comm.* Communication of
Dr. D.J. Corrigan Feb. 1859
H.C. 1862 xii (95).
31. *Eleventh rep. ILI*, app. F.
32. *Journ. Ment. Sc.* iv (1858),
p. 257.
33. Insp. lun. papers memo. to
lord-lieutenant 12-4-1882.
34 Burdett, *Hospitals and Asylums of the World* i, p. 256.
35 *Twenty third rep. ILA* 1873,
app. H.; *General Rules and
Regulations for the Management of District Lunatic
Asylums in Ireland 1894.*
36. Insp. Lun. papers memo.
J. Nugent to Sir Robert
Hamilton 10-8-1885.
37. *ibid*, memo. to lord lieutenant 12-4-1882.
38. *Twenty third rep. ILI*, p.
104.
39. Memo. 12-4-1882.
40. *Thirty second rep. ILI*, pp.
14-22, 174-177.
41. *ibid.* p. 20.
42. Insp. Lun. papers memo. to
lord-lieutenant from Mitchell
and Holmes 21-3-1885.
43. Memo 10-8-1885.
44. Insp. Lun. papers. Mitchell
to Holmes 8-3-1892.
45. *Journ. Ment. Sc.* xxxvi
(1890), pp. 309-310.
46. Report to lord-lieutenant
15-12-1891.
47. *First and second reps.
comm. lun. admin. Ire.* 1890,
pp. 46-47.
48. *Forty second rep. ILI*, p. 10.
49. Letters, *Freeman's Journ.*
George Kidd 25-4-1892;
Connolly Norman 26-4-1892;
Archibald Jacob 13-4-1892.
50. 1 & 2 Geo iv, cap. 23, ss.
3-5.
51. *Rep. lunatic poor* 1843 q
170; *Rules* 1843.
52. 30 and 31 Vic., c. 118, s.3.
53. *Hansard* cxliii (1856), pars.
1759-1766.
54. *Lunatic poor (Ire.) correspondence* ... 1844, p. 4
H.C. 1844 xliii (233).
55. *Journ. Ment. Sc.* iv, (1858),
p. 271.
56. *Rep. lunatic poor* 1843 q
481.
57. *ibid* q 365.
58. *Report comms. enq. asy.
Ire.* 1858 pt. 1, p. 8.
59. Larcom papers ms 7775.
60. *Twenty first rep. ILI*, app.
c. 26.
61. *Twenty third rep. ILI*, p.
148.
62. *Twenty fifth rep. ILI*, p. 9;
app. E. 27.
63. *Thirty-second rep. ILI*, p. 9.
64. *Thirty-seventh rep. ILI*, p. 14

Chapter 8

1. Scull, *Museums of Madness*, p. 238.
2. *Twenty second report ILI*, p. 6.
3. *Tenth report ILI*, app. no. 9; *forty second report*, table xiv.
4. *Eighth report ILI*, p. 25.
5. *Ninth report ILI*, p. 12.
6. *Forty second report ILI*, table xiii; *forty third report*, app. G.
7. Scull, *Madhouses, Mad Doctors and Madmen*, pp. 313-330.
8. Burdett *op. cit.* i, p. 161.
9. *Forty third report*, p. 5 and app. G.
10. *ibid*, app. G, p. 209.
11. Drapes, *On the Alleged Increase of Insanity in Ireland*; *Forty third report ILI*. pp. 5, 6, 194 and app. G.
12. *An Account of Ireland Political and Statistical* i, p. 729.
13. O'Brien, *Economic History of Ireland*, p. 351.
14. *Eighth report ILI*, p. 24.
15. *Tenth report ILI*, app. 10; *forty second report*, table xiii; *forty third report*, app. G.
16. *Supplement to fifty-fourth report ILI*, p. xxi.
17. O'Hare and Walsh, *Activities of Irish Psychiatric Hospitals and Units 1982*, table 4.
18. Chapetz and Demone, *Alcoholism and Society*, pp. 33-61; Goodwin and Guze, *Psychiatric Diagnosis*, p. 20.
19. Vaillant, *The Natural History of Alcoholism*, p. 3.
20. 42 & 43 Vic. c. 19; 51 & 52 Vic. c. 19; 61 & 62 Vic. c. 60.
21. *Hansard*, third series ccxliii (1879), par. 1385.
22. 42 & 43 Vic. c. 19, s. 10.
23. *Thirteenth report, Inspector for Ireland under the Inebriates Acts* 1917, table iii.
24. 61 & 62 Vic. c. 60.
25. Tim Kelly, Ennis County Jail in *North Munster Antiquarian Journal* xvi (1973-4), p. 69.
26. *Annual Reports 1904-1970 Inspector under Inebriates Acts*.
27. Burdett *op. cit.*, p. 122.
28. *Sixth report ILI*, p. 19; *eighth report*, pp. 12-13.
29. *Eighth report*, p. 12.
30. *First report ILI*, app. 1; *sixth report*, app. 1.
31. *Report comms. enq.* 1858 pt. 2 qq 184-186; *Nineteenth report ILI*, p. 11.
32. *Journ. Ment. Sc.* vii (1861) pp. 59-79.
33. *ibid* vi (1860), pp. 167-178.
34. *ibid* vi, pp. 179-198.
35. *ibid* vi, pp. 197-198; *Dublin Quart. Journ. Med. Sc.* xxx, pp. 421-423; *Tenth report ILI*, p. 15.
36. See Bowen, *The Protestant Crusade in Ireland* 1800-1870.
37. Handlin, *Bostons Immigrants 1790-1865; A Study in Acculturation*, p. 126.

38. *Fifty fourth rep. ILI* supplement, pp. xxiii-xxviii.
39. Ross, *Statistics of Insanity in New South Wales with Reference to the Census of 1891*, p. 87.
40. *Fifty fourth report ILI* supp. p. xxviii.
41. *Annual Report Cork District Lunatic Asylum* 1909, pp. 13-14.
42. *Thirty seventh report ILI*, p. 6.
43. *Forty third report ILI*, app. G.
44. *Fifty fourth report ILI* supplement, p. xxiii.
45. *Ann. Report Cork D.L.A.* 1909, p. 14.
46. *Freeman's Journal* 14-7-1899; *Tuam Herald* 3-7-1909.
47. *Fifty fourth report ILI* Suppl.
48. Carstairs and Kennedy, Social Science in relation to Psychiatry in *Companion to Psychiatric Studies* sec. ed., p. 17.
49. Schrier, *Ireland and the American Emigration 1850-1900*, p. 21.
50. Kennedy, *The Irish: Emigration, Marriage and Fertility*, pp. 88-93.
51. *ibid*, pp. 66-85.
52. *ibid*, pp. 75-76.
53. Fallows, *Irish Americans: Identity and Assimilation*, p. 32; Wittke, *The Irish in America*, pp. 62-63.
54. Thernstrom, *Social Mobility in a Nineteenth Century City*, pp. 18-27, 150-152.
55. Wittke, op. cit p. 44; Fallows, op. cit. p. 33.
56. Biddiss, *Images of Race*, p. 29.
57. Kingsley, *His Letters and Memories of His Life* ii, p. 107.
58. Wittke, op. cit. p. 46.
59. Thernstrom, pp. 25-26.

Chapter 9

1. Hodder, *The Life and Work of the Seventh Earl of Shaftesbury* iii, pp. 118-119.
2. *Rep. insp. gen. pris. on asy.* 1843, app. 3, pars. 8, 10, 28.
3. Tuke *op. cit.*, p. 485.
4. *Standing Rules and Regulations of the Royal Irish Constabulary 6th Ed.* 1911, p. 239.
5. *Nineteenth rep. ILI*, p. 16.
6. *Journ. Ment. Sc.* xxi, p. 107.
7. *Eighth rep*, p. 15.
8. *Rep. comms. enq. lun. asy. Ire.* 1858 pt. 1, pp. 13-16.
9. *Dublin Quart. Journ. Med. Sc.* xxxii (1861), pp. 337-380.
10. *Daily Express* (Dublin) 14-10-1858; *Evening Post* 19-11-1858; *The Nation* 20-11-1858.
11. *Twenty-third rep. ILI*, p. 209 and app. H lxiv.
12. *General rules etc. 1894*, lv.
13. *Rep. insp. gen. pris. on asy.* 1843, app. 3.
14. *First rep. ILI*, p. 17.

15. *Short Hints and observations on the Arrangement and Management of Lunatic Asylums.*
16. *Gen. rules etc. 1894.*
17. Blake, *Defects in the Moral Treatment of Insanity in the Public Lunatic Asylums of Ireland*, p. 99.
18. *Sel. comm* 1843, p. xxiv.
19. *Comms. enq.* 1848 pt. 2 qq 1741, 1742, 3072, 3073, 3086.
20. Blake *op. cit.*, p. 85.
21. Inspectors of lunacy papers; report to lord-lieut. Dec. 1891.
22. Burdett *op. cit.* i, p. 260.
23. *Dublin Quart. Journ. Med.* Sc. xxxii (1861) pp. 375-376.
24. Burdett *op. cit.* i, p. 644.
25. Finnane *op. cit.*, p. 181.
26. *Eighteenth rep. ILI*, app. B. 19.
27. *Twenty second rep. ILI*, p. 10.
28. *Thirty sixth rep. ILI*, p. 13; *forty eighth rep.* p. 13.
29. *Forty second rep. ILI*, pp. 138-140.
30. *Comms. inq.* 1858, pt. 2, qq 1741, 1750-1760, 2137-2158.
31. Joseph Lalor, *On the Use of Education and Training in the Treatment of the Insane in Public Lunatic Asylums* 1878; JSSISI vii, pp. 361-373.
32. Burdett *op. cit.* i, p. 252.
33. *Thirty sixth report ILI*, p. 14; Tuke *op. cit.*, p. 438.
34. Norman, The Family Care of the Insane in *Medical Press and Circular* 29 Nov. and 6 Dec. 1905.
35. The Domestic Treatment of the Insane in *Trans. Royal Acad. Med. Ire.* xiii, p. 3, 1896.
36. Wynter and Granville, *The Borderlines of Insanity and other Papers*, pp. 124-131; *New Catholic Encyclopedia* iv, p. 1130.
37. *Forty fourth rep. ILI*, p. 102.
38. Norman, *Family Care of Persons of Unsound Mind* 1903, p. 16.
39. *Twenty first rep. ILI*, p. 8; *forty second rep.*, table xix.
40. *Forty first rep*, p. 7.
41. Robins, *The Lost Children*, pp. 157-173.
42. *Seventeenth rep. L.G.B.I.*, p. 6.
43. *Ninth rep. ILI*, pp. 10-11.
44. *Fifty fifth rep. ILI*, pp. lxvi-lxvii.
45. Burdett *op. cit.* i, pp. 242-246.

Chapter 10

1. Burdett *op. cit.* i, p. 575.
2. 1 and 2 Geo. c. 33, s. 5; *Sel. comm. 1843* q 170; *Rep. insp. gen. pris. 1843*, app. 3.
3. 1 Vic. c. 27, s. 1; Hancock,

On the assimilation of the Law in England, Scotland and Ireland as to the care of lunatics and their property in *JSSISI* viii, pp. 79-82.

4. *Sel. comm. 1843*, p. xii.

5. *ibid*, p. viii.

6. *Hansard* lxxvi (1844), pars. 619-622.

7. 8 and 9 Vic. c. 107, s. 10.

8. 30 and 31 Vic. c. 118, ss. 10, 11.

9. *Twenty fourth rep. ILI*, p. 10.

10. *ibid*, app. E.2; *First and second reps. comm. lun. adm. (Ire) 1890-91*, pp. 38-42 H.C. 1891 (739), xxxvi.

11. *Hansard* cclx (1881), pars. 802-823.

12. 38 and 39 Vic. c. 67, s. 16.

13. *Fifty fourth rep. ILI*, p. 5.

14. Reps. 1890-91, pp. 33-43; 53 and 54 Vic. c. 5.

15. 39 and 40 Geo. III c. 94; 1 and 2 Vic. c. 14.

16. 1 and 1 Geo. IV. c. 33, ss. 16-18.

17. 1 Vic. c. 27, ss. 2, 3.

18. Jones, *Lunacy Law and Conscience* 1744-1845, pp. 209-213.

19. *Ann. rep. ins. gen. pris. on lun. poor 1844*, p. 6.

20. *Rep. comm. lun. poor Ire. 1843 q.* 123.

21. 8 and 9 Vic. c. 107, s. i; *Pauper Lunatics (Ireland); copies of corresp. etc. 1844.* H.C. 1844 (603), xliii.

22. Tuke *op. cit.*, p. 268-271.

23. *Second ann. rep. ILI*, pp. 9-11.

24. *Fifth ann. rep. ILI*, p. 10; *eighth ann. rep.*, p. 19; *twenty fifth ann. rep.* p. 18.

25. Insp. lun. pap. rep. comm. enq., Dec. 1891.

26. 38 and 39 Vic. c. 67; 46 and 47 Vic. c. 38; 47 and 48 Vic. c. 64.

27. 1 Edw. 7. c. 17; 4 and 5 Geo. 5. c. 58.

28. *Adaptation of Enactments Act 1922* (2 of 1922); *Ministers and Secretaries Act 1924* (16 of 1924).

29. *Criminal Justice Act 1960* (27 of 1960), ss. 3, 4. 8.

30. Carte, *The Life of the Duke of Ormond* iv, pp. 95-100; Abraham, *The Law and the Practice of Lunacy in Ireland*, pp. 2-6.

31. 17 Edw. c. 9.

32. Carte, *A History of the Life of James Duke of Ormonde* i, p. 49.

33. Carte, *The Life . . .*, p. 95-100.

34. Abraham *op. cit.*, p. 49; 15 Ch. 1. c. 53; 6 Geo. 4. c. 53; 1 Will. 4. c. 65; 5 and 6 Will. 4. c. 17; 15 and 16 Vic. c. 48.

35. 5 and 6 Vic. c. 123, ss. 13, 38; Insp. Lun. Pap. R.W. Holmes to Arthur Mitchell 24-2-1892.

36. Insp. Lun. Pap. memo. of Lord Ashbourne and associated corresp. June 1892.

37. *Dictionary of National Biography* xiv, pp. 947-949; Tuke *op. cit.*, pp. 431-441.

38. 34 Vic. c. 22.

39. 43 and 44 Vic. c. 39.

40. *Dictionary of National Bi-*

ography 1912-1921, p. 209.

41. Memo. June 1892.

42. *First and sec. reps. comm.*

lun. admin. 1890-1891, pp. 49-52.

43. Memo. June 1892; 1 Edw. 7.

Chapter 11

1. Michael Craft ed., *Tredgold's Mental Retardation* 12th ed., p. 3.

2. Maloney and Ward, *Mental Retardation and Modern Society*, p. 9.

3. Maloney and Ward, p. 19; Cytryn and Lourie, Mental Retardation in *Comprehensive Text book of Psychiatry* i, pp. 1158-59.

4. *General rules* etc., 1843, rule 4.

5. *Rep. insp. gen. on asy.* 1844, p. 5.

6. Correspondence books Joseph Burke; circ letter 25-11-1842; *First rep. comms. cond. poor Ire.* 1835, app. B., pp. 388-389.

7. *Sel. comm.* 1843, p. xxv.

8. *Rep. insp. gen.* 1844, app. 5.

9. *First rep. ILI*, p. 11.

10. *Comms. inq. lun. asy. Ire.* 1858 pt. 1, p. 19.

11. *Twelfth rep. ILI*, apps. B.2 and C.9; *forty second rep. ILI*, app. D.

12. *Comms. inq. 1858* pt. 2, qq 733-744; *tenth rep. ILI*, app. F; *Union Workhouses (Ireland) (Sick Persons).*

13. Sigerson, The Law and the Lunatic in JSSISI ix, p. 26.

14. Tuke *op. cit.*, pp. 301-302; Cytryn and Lourie *op. cit.*, pp. 1158-59; Apley ed. *Care of the Handicapped Child*,

p. 17.

15. Cytryn and Lourie, op. cit. p. 1158.

16. *Dublin quar. journ. med. sc.* xxxix, pp. 174-192.

17. Pim, On the necessity of State Provision for the Education of the Deaf, Dumb, Blind and Imbecile in *JSSISI* iv (1868), pp. 26-41.

18. Kidd, *An appeal on behalf of the Idiotic and Imbecile Children of Ireland 1866.*

19. *Proposed Institution for the Training etc. of Children. Proceedings of Meetings in Belfast* Feb. 1867. Stewarts Hospital papers.

20. Widdess, *The Richmond, Whitworth and Hardwicke Hospitals. St. Laurences Hospital 1772-1972*, pp. 73, 93, 94; *Ninth rep. ILI*, p. 22.

21. *Reports of Committee and Rules for Admission of Pupils and Patients* 1869-1870. Minutes of sub-committee July 1868-April 1870.

22. *Dublin Evening Mail* 15 Feb. 1869.

23. Minutes of sub-com. 16-2-1869, 17-2-1869.

24. Annual reports of management committee 1870-1880.

25. Jones op. cit., pp. 184-185; 49 Vic. c. 25.

26. *Rep. poor law and lun. inq.* (Ire) 1879, pp. lxxxvi-c.

(2239) xxxi, pp. lxxxvi-c.

27. *Sixty first rep. ILI*, p. xxxiii.
28. 41 and 42 Vic. c. 60.
29. *Forty first rep. ILI*, p. 19.
30. 61 and 62 Vic. c. 37, ss. 9, 76 and part 3.
31. *Rep. comm. sick and dest. poor* 1927, pp. 105-106.
32. *ibid*, p. 106; *fifty fourth rep. ILI*, p. xliii.
33. 61 and 62 Vic. c. 37, s. 76.
34. *Rep. vice regal comm. poor law Ire.* i, p. 38.
35. *Sixty fourth rep. ILI*, app. F.
36. *Tredgold's Mental Retardation*, p. 4; Gelder, Gath, Mayou, *Oxford Textbook of Psychiatry*, p. 687.
37. 62 and 63 Vic. c. 32.
38. *Rep. comm. care feeble minded* viii, pp. 417-470
39. 17 and 18 Geo. 5, c. 23.
40. *Rep.* pp. 432-433.
41. 3 and 4 Geo. 5, c. 28.

Chapter 12

1. *Sixty fourth rep. ILI*, pp. x-xi.
2. Mora, Historical and Theoretical Trends in Psychiatry in *Comprehensive Textbook of Psychiatry*, pp. 56-59; Goodwin and Guze, *Psychiatric Diagnosis* sec. ed., pp. 4-5.
3. O'Shea and Falvey, A History of St. Brendan's Hospital Dublin in *Psychiatric Nursing* Autumn 1984, p. 32.
4. 61 and 62 Vic. c. 37.
5. Collins, The Evolutions of County Government in *Administration* i, 2, p. 80.
6. *Sligo Independent* 27-6-1908.
7. Robinson, *Memories; Wise and Otherwise,* pp. 131-132.
8. 61 and 62 Vic. c. 37, ss. 58.76.
9. *Sixty fourth rep. ILI*, p. xi.
10. *Sixty sixth rep. ILI*, p. xvi.
11. *Irish Times* 27-5-1909; *Free-man's Journal* 7-6-1909; *Irish Independent* 7-6-1909.
12. Rowland, *Lloyd George,* p. 202.
13. *Rep. comm. dest. poor* 1927, p. 99.
14. Vol. viii part xiii, p. 448.
15. H.C. 1906 (3202), lii.
16. H.C. 1909 (4630), xxxviii.
17. *Report vice-regal comm.* vol 3, p. 992.
18. *Mins. evid.* qq 16144, 1768, 19108-19110.
19. *Report*, vol 1, pp. 37.40
20. *Mins. evid.* qq 28441-28533; appendices pp. 256-259.
21. Millar, *Church, State and Nation in Ireland 1898-1921*, pp. 268-292.
22. *Journ. Med. Sc.* liii, (220), pp. 164-165.
23. *Report royal comm; report on Ireland*, par. 320.
24. Robinson *op. cit.*, pp. 212-317.
25. *ibid*, p. 217.

26. *Sixty eighth rep. ILI*, pp. vi, vii, xviii-xxi.
27. *Thirty fifth ann. rep. Enniscorthy asy.*, p. 15.
28. *Report Derry asy. 1910*, app. xxvi; *Report Sligo asy.* 1910, p. 23; *Irish Times* 7-8-1911.
29. Granville, *Care and Cure of the Insane*, p. 99.
30. *Irish Independent* 23-11-1907, 21-1-1908;*Irish Times* 27-1-1908.
31. 30 and 31 Vic. c. 118.
32. *Rep. and evid. sel. comm. asy. officers superannuation 1909*, q 286.
33. *ibid* q 3; *Irish Times* 25-9-1911.
34. *Irish Times* 25-9-1911.
35. 9 Edw. 7. c. 48; 8 and 9 Geo. 5. c. 33; 9 and 10 Geo. 5. c. 67.
36. *Irish Times* 27-3-1911.
37. Daniel Murphy unpublished account p. 14.
38. *Nenagh News* 1-1-1919, 8-1-1919.
39. *Nenagh Guardian* 14-6-1919, 13-9-1919, 20-9-1919.
40. Murphy ed., *Tumbling Walls*, p. 40.
41. Daniel Murphy *op. cit.*; *ann. rep. IMH 1924*, pp. 16-17.
42. Daniel Murphy, pp. 43-47.
43. *Ann. rep. Derry asy. 1910*, p. 39.
44. *Ann. rep. IMH 1925*, pp. 9-14.
45. 9 and 10 Geo. 5. c. 96.
46. Information provided by An Bord Altranais.
47. *Rep. comm. relief sick. dest. poor* 1927, par. 478.
48. *Ann. rep. IMH 1951*, p. 27.
49. *Tumbling Walls*, p. 44.
50. *Local Government (Temporary Provisions) Act 1923*
51. *Ann. rep. IMH 1923*; *first rep ILNI 1924*.
52. *Local Government Act 1925* s. 79.
53. *Dail Eireann: Parliamentary Debates* ii, par. 485.
54. Boyd-Barrett, Modern Psychotherapy and our Asylums in *Studies* xiii (1924), pp. 29-43.
55. *Rep. comm. relief sick dest. poor*, pars. 362-515.
56. Par. 416.
57. Par. 422.
58. Pars. 440-443.
59. Pars. 428-436.
60. Pars. 432-434.
61. Pars. 447-470.

Chapter 13

1. *Public Charitable Hospitals (Amendment) Act 1931*; *Public Hospitals Act 1933*.
2. *Rep. comm. enq. mental illness*, app. 1.
3. *Rep. IMH 1955*, p. 2.
4. *Rep. IMH 1960*, p. 10.
5. Sheehan and de Barra, *Ospideïl na nEireann* 1930-1955, pp. 22-62.

6. *New Catholic Ency.* i, pp 470-473.
7. McKenna, John Cidade, A Case for Treatment? in *Caritas* 46 (38), p. 31.
8. Cooney, *A Service for the Mentally Handicapped.*
9. Report by Dr L.S. Clifford on investigations of mental deficiency and sane epilepsy May 1943, unpublished.
10. *Rep. services for mentally handicapped* 1980, pars. 4.20, 4.21.
11. *Rep. comm. inq. mental handicap*, pp. 34-45.
12. 20 and 21 Geo. 5. c. 23; 22 and 23 Geo 5. c. 15 (Northern Ireland).
13. *Mental Treatment Act 1945 Ministers and Secretaries (Amendement) Act 1946.*
14. *Mental Treatment Act*, part xiv.
15. *ibid* ss. 96, 97, 189, 217, 220-222, 236, 237, 250, 266.
16. *ibid*, part xviii.
17. Kennedy, Physical Methods of Treatment in *Companion to Psychiatric Studies* sec. ed., pp. 535-548; Mora *op. cit.*, pp. 68-70; Jones *op. cit.*, pp. 291-297.
18. Maudsley, *Body and Mind* rev. ed., 1873.
19. Viney, *Mental Illness*, p. 10.
20. *Health Act 1953.*
21. *Rep. IMH 1961-62*, pp. 10-11.
22. *Report IMH 1961-62*, p. 13.
23. *A Hospital Plan for England and Wales* 1962; US Joint Commission on Mental Illness and Health, *Action for Mental Health*, 1961.
24. McKeown, 'The concept of a balanced hospital community' in *Lancet* i (1958), pp. 701-704.
25. *Report IMH 1961-62*, p. 5.
26. Walsh, *The 1963 Irish Psychiatric Hospital Census*, table v.
27. *ibid*, pp. 11-13; O'Hare and Walsh, *Irish Psychiatric Hospitals and Units Census 1981*, pp. 10-11.
28. O'Hare and Walsh, *Activities of Irish Psychiatric Hospitals and Units 1965-1969*, tables 10-19, 25-28.
29. Dean and others, First admissions to psychiatric hospitals in south-east England in 1976 among immigrants from Ireland in *British Medical Journal* vol. 282, June 1981.
30. *Planning for the Future*, p. 2.
31. *Department of Health, Statistical Report* 1984, Table 16.
32. *Planning for the Future*, table 4.
33. Gregg, *The Welfare State*, pp. 6-7.
34. 14 and 15 Vic. c. 68.
35. *Planning for the Future*, tables 10-16.
36. O'Hare and Walsh, *Activites of Irish Psychiatric Hospitals and Units 1982*, table 23.

Epilogue

1. *Comm. enq. mental handicap 1965; comm. enq. mental illness 1966.*
2. *Health Act 1970.*
3. *Statistical information relevant to the health services 1984,* sect. E.
4. *The Psychiatric Services: Planning for the Future 1984.*
5. *Health (Mental Services) Act, 1981.*
6. *Statistical information etc.,* sect. F.
7. *Reports: Dail Eireann, Vol. 363 (6) par. 1334.*

Index